HEALING
Gourmet®
Eat to Beat
Diabetes

D0974826

HEALING

Gourmet®

Eat to Beat Diabetes

THE EDITORS OF HEALING GOURMET WITH

Paresh Dandona, M.D., FACP,

Melissa Ohlson, M.S., RD, and Ana Machado, CEC

McGraw·Hill

New York   Chicago   San Francisco   Lisbon   London   Madrid   Mexico City
Milan   New Delhi   San Juan   Seoul   Singapore   Sydney   Toronto

Library of Congress Cataloging-in-Publication Data

Healing gourmet, eat to beat diabetes / with Paresh Dandona, Melissa Ohlson, and Ana C. Machado.
p.   cm.
Includes bibliographical references and index.
ISBN 0-07-145755-0 (alk. paper)
1. Diabetes—Diet therapy—Popular works.   I. Title: Eat to beat diabetes.
II. Dandona, Paresh.   III. Ohlson, Melissa.   IV. Machado, Ana C.
V. Healing gourmet.

RC662.H42   2006
616.4′620654—dc22   2005009867

2 3 4 5 6 7 8 9 0   FGR/FGR   0 9 8 7 6

ISBN 0-07-145755-0

Interior design by Monica Baziuk

McGraw-Hill books are available at special quantity discounts to use as premiums and sales promotions, or for use in corporate training programs. For more information, please write to the Director of Special Sales, Professional Publishing, McGraw-Hill, Two Penn Plaza, New York, NY 10121-2298. Or contact your local bookstore.

This book is printed on acid-free paper.

This book is dedicated to those living with diabetes.

Contents

Acknowledgments

THIS BOOK IS brought to you with the assistance and knowledge of medical, culinary, and nutrition experts from across the nation, as well as the diligent work of countless scientists worldwide who helped us to translate research into recipes in our mission to educate individuals on the link between diet and disease. Healing Gourmet would like to thank the following people for their contribution.

A very special thanks to our editor Natasha Graf for her attention to detail and function as catalyst for many of the concepts presented in the book, as well as to our project editor, Nancy Hall, for her diligence in the preparation of the final manuscript.

Our medical, nutrition, and culinary editors: Thanks to Dr. Paresh Dandona for his thorough review and guidance; to Melissa Ohlson for her speedy and meticulous work on recipe analysis, meal planning, and nutritional review; and Ana Machado for her culinary expertise and recipe testing to ensure our recipes deliver as much taste as they do health.

Our publisher: Thanks to McGraw-Hill for their commitment to delivering high-quality information to the public, including many of the educational textbooks that spurred the development of this company.

Our affiliations: Thanks to the fine institutions that bring us these editors, including Kaleida Health, Cleveland Clinic Foundation, and Florida Culinary Institute.

Our associates and family: Thanks to Guy Gelin, and our families and friends for their continuing support of the Healing Gourmet project.

Introduction

HEALING GOURMET BEGAN with a mission to educate people on the link between diet and disease. As part of a series, this book is meant to provide useful information on eating to beat diabetes through sound nutritional principles. We bring the "clinic" together with the "kitchen," to help you deliciously make the most of your health through the latest discoveries. Quite simply, Healing Gourmet translates research to recipes, making your kitchen a healing haven.

In this book, we will help you to understand the basic principles of diabetes and how your diet can help to manage your disease and prevent complications. Chapters 1 and 2 focus on the basics of diabetes: how the disease works, your diagnosis, monitoring your condition, complications, and the lifestyle changes to help you take control. In Chapter 3 we address metabolic syndrome, insulin resistance, the factors of inflammation, and how your favorite fruits and vegetables can protect you. In Chapter 4, we'll give you the skinny on fat and the truth about carbohydrates. Then we'll introduce you to your diabetes-beating arsenal of phytonutrients and antioxidants (Chapter 5) and to the delicious foods (Chapter 6) and herbs and spices (Chapter 7) where you can find these nutrients.

Of course, we'll help you to sleuth out the healthiest products at the grocery in Chapter 8, help you plan your diabetes-beating meals in Chapter 9, and give you fifty great recipes to get started in Chapter 10. Don't forget to visit our website, healing gourmet.com, for the latest research and more diabetes-beating recipes!

IMPORTANT DISCLAIMER: *The information in this book cannot replace the advice of your physician or health-care team. Always consult with your doctor or dietitian before making any changes in diet.*

Letter from the Editor

CAN SOMETHING AS delicious as a Berry Tart with Cinnamon Oat Crust really help to balance blood sugar? This is just one of the questions we set out to answer nearly five years ago with the creation of our company. Dedicated solely to helping the public make better food choices to prevent disease, Healing Gourmet brings you sound, scientific evidence and practical solutions to help you take control of your health.

Our recipe for health is simple. First, we take a disease-fighting dose of research collected from the National Library of Medicine on your favorite foods, compounds in foods, and their effects on disease. Right at this very moment, scientists are hard at work analyzing nutrients in foods for their beneficial effects on blood sugar, their cholesterol-lowering capacity, and their cancer-fighting action. Other researchers are poring over data from population studies to give us clues to why disease rates are lower in other countries where their diets differ greatly from those in the United States. Together, this research in the New Nutritional Frontier acts as the foundation—the first ingredient—in a disease-fighting mix. To help us in this research, we are extremely fortunate to have the assistance of Paresh Dandona, M.D., as a contributor. As a professor of medicine and pharmacology and head of the division of endocrinology at State University of New York, Dr. Dandona has done extensive research in the antioxidative and anti-inflammatory effects of insulin and insulin sensitizers and the effects of macronutrients. The second step in our recipe for health is incorporating these scientific findings with culinary finesse to whip up mouth-watering recipes and easy-to-use meal plans so you can make the most of the latest nutritional breakthroughs. For this task, we are also lucky to have the expertise and nutritional analysis of Melissa Ohlson, M.S., R.D.—the nutrition projects coordinator, preventive cardiology & rehabilitation at the Cleveland Clinic Heart Center—and the culinary expertise in testing and creating recipes of Ana Machado, C.E.C.—a chef instructor at Florida Culinary Institute. More on these amazing contributors is listed in the next section.

Don't forget to visit us on the Web at healinggourmet.com and look for us on television this fall debuting on the Healthy Living Channel. Enjoy these books in good health and remember to *eat your medicine!*

    —KELLEY LUNSFORD
    Editor-in-Chief
    Chairman, President & C.E.O.

About the Contributors

Medical Editor

Paresh Dandona, M.B.B.S., D.Phil., FRCP, FACP, FACE, FACC, is professor of medicine and pharmacology and head of the division of endocrinology at State University of New York, Buffalo, New York. He is head of the division of endocrinology, Kaleida Health, Buffalo, New York, and the director and founder of the Diabetes-Endocrinology Center of Western New York. Dr. Dandona is a past Rhodes Scholar trained in endocrinology at the University of Oxford. His research interests include insulin resistance and atherosclerosis, the antioxidative and anti-inflammatory effects of insulin and insulin sensitizers, and the effects of macronutrients. He has authored more than four hundred peer reviewed scientific publications and is the editor in chief of the journal *Metabolic Syndrome and Related Disorders.*

Nutrition Editor

Melissa Ohlson, M.S., RD, is the nutrition projects coordinator, Preventive Cardiology & Rehabilitation at the Cleveland Clinic Heart Center. Her broad scope of work includes medical nutrition therapy, coordination of nutrition activities at the clinic, development of online nutrition programs, and involvement with the *Cooking for Your Heart* culinary program series in association with the Cleveland Clinic. Melissa is also a personal trainer and a nutrition consultant.

Culinary Editor

Ana Machado, CEC, is a chef instructor at Florida Culinary Institute in West Palm Beach, Florida. Her devotion to healthy, nutritionally balanced spa cuisine led her to California's Wine Country where she worked as an executive chef in three restaurants in and around Carmel. She has also worked as a private chef to many VIPs and has catered for the likes of Andrew Lloyd Weber, Alice Waters, Clint Eastwood, and Michael Douglas.

HEALING *Gourmet*
Eat to Beat Diabetes

Understanding Diabetes

DIABETES IS A DISEASE in which blood glucose levels are above normal. People with diabetes have problems converting food to energy. After a meal, food is broken down into a sugar called *glucose*, which is carried by the blood to cells throughout the body. Cells use the hormone *insulin*, made in the pancreas, to help them process blood glucose into energy. Insulin is secreted when glucose from a meal enters the bloodstream. The only way cells in the body are able to process glucose into energy is through insulin. Without it, the blood levels of glucose continue to rise, leading to damage of cells in the body.

How Diabetes Works and Its Different Types

After eating a meal, food is digested and broken down for absorption. As these compounds are absorbed, they are released for transport into the bloodstream. Foods are broken down into a variety of nutrients, such as fats, proteins, and carbohydrates. Foods that contain naturally occurring or added sugars and carbohydrates break down into glucose. As they are released into the bloodstream after digestion, blood glucose levels rise. As blood glucose rises, the pancreas is signaled to secrete insulin. Although insulin is constantly being secreted in small amounts, eating triggers an increase in the insulin that is released. The insulin attaches to cells and allows the glucose to enter, as a key unlocks a door and lets you in. The glucose provides the necessary energy for cells to carry out their biological duties. When we take in more glucose than our cells need for energy, the excess glucose is sent to the liver for storage. This stored glucose can be used for energy when our blood glucose levels fall lower than they should—such as between meals, when we are exercising for long periods, or when we fast.

As sugar is removed from the bloodstream through this process, blood glucose levels drop and, in turn, insulin decreases. When we begin to eat again, the liver is signaled to halt the release of its sugar reserve, and blood glucose levels return to a normal range. Now armed with this information, we can look more closely at the various types of diabetes.

Type 1 Diabetes

Type 1 diabetes, which was formerly called juvenile diabetes or insulin-dependent diabetes, is usually first diagnosed in children, teenagers, or young adults. In this form, the beta cells of the pancreas no longer make insulin because the body's immune system has attacked and destroyed them. Treatment for type 1 diabetes includes taking insulin shots or using an insulin pump, making wise food choices, exercising regularly, and controlling blood pressure and cholesterol.

Type 2 Diabetes

Type 2 diabetes, which was formerly called adult-onset or non-insulin-dependent diabetes (NIDDM), is the most common form of diabetes. People can develop type 2 diabetes at any age, even during childhood when the cells in the body do not use insulin properly. Eventually, the pancreas cannot make enough insulin for the body's needs. As a result, the amount of glucose in the blood increases while the cells are starved of energy. Over the years, high blood glucose damages nerves and blood vessels, leading to complications such as heart disease, stroke, blindness, kidney disease, nerve problems, gum infections, and amputation. We will discuss the complications of diabetes in more detail later in the chapter.

With type 2 diabetes, cells become numb to the action of insulin. This form of diabetes usually begins with *insulin resistance*, a condition in which cells in the body fat, muscle, and liver cells do not use insulin properly. When cells become resistant to insulin, the level of glucose in the blood stays high. At first, the pancreas keeps up with the added demand by producing more insulin. Over time, however, it loses the ability to secrete enough insulin in response to meals.

Because glucose cannot enter the cells, the cells then think that there is no glucose in the blood. As a result, the cells send a signal to the liver, prompting it to release any stored glucose it has into the bloodstream. As the body tries to compensate and shuttle glucose into the cells, the pancreas secretes more insulin. Because insulin isn't able to perform its function, blood glucose levels can rise unchecked. As glucose levels in the blood increase, they slowly damage other cells in the body. If not controlled over the long term, this can lead to complications such as heart disease, kidney disease, and amputation. High glucose levels in the blood also escape through the kidneys, bringing with it water leading to dehydration. Severe dehydration can result in *hyperosmolic nonketotic diabetic coma*, a life-threatening complication.

Being overweight and inactive increases the chances of developing type 2 diabetes. Treatment includes taking diabetes medicines, making wise food choices, exercising regularly, and controlling blood pressure and cholesterol.

Gestational Diabetes

Some women develop *gestational diabetes* during the late stages of pregnancy. Although this form of diabetes usually goes away after the baby is born, a woman who has had it is more likely to develop type 2 diabetes later in life. Gestational diabetes is caused by the hormones of pregnancy or a shortage of insulin.

Risk Factors for Type 2 Diabetes

You can do a lot to lower your chances of getting type 2 diabetes, especially with your diet, which is why we offer so many helpful recipes and meal plans to get you started on your way to good health. Exercising regularly, reducing fat and calorie intake, and losing weight can all help you reduce your risk. Lowering blood pressure and cholesterol levels also help you stay healthy. Your risk for diabetes is increased if:

* You are overweight
* You are 45 years old or older
* You have a parent, brother, or sister with diabetes
* Your family background is African American, Native American, Asian American, Pacific Islander, or Hispanic American/Latino
* You have had gestational diabetes or have given birth to at least one baby weighing more than nine pounds
* Your blood pressure is 140/90 or higher, or you have been told that you have high blood pressure
* Your cholesterol levels are not normal (the HDL or "good" cholesterol is 35 or lower, or your triglyceride level is 250 or higher)
* You are fairly inactive (exercise fewer than three times a week)

❖ You have been diagnosed with *prediabetes*, also called *impaired glucose tolerance* (*IGT*) or *impaired fasting glucose* (*IFG*) (Prediabetes is a condition in which your blood glucose—or blood sugar—levels are higher than normal but not high enough for a diagnosis of diabetes. Those with prediabetes are likely to develop type 2 diabetes within ten years, unless they take steps to prevent or delay diabetes. The results of a study called the Diabetes Prevention Program showed that modest weight loss and regular exercise can prevent or delay type 2 diabetes.)

Warning Signs

Many people have no signs or symptoms. Symptoms can also be so mild that you might not even notice them. More than five million people in the United States have type 2 diabetes and do not know it. Here is what to look for:

❖ Increased thirst
❖ Increased hunger
❖ Fatigue
❖ Increased urination, especially at night
❖ Weight gain
❖ Blurred vision
❖ Sores that do not heal

Sometimes people have symptoms but do not suspect diabetes. They delay scheduling a checkup because they do not feel sick. Many people do not find out they have the disease until they have diabetes complications, such as blurry vision or heart trouble. It is important to find out early if you have diabetes because early treatment can prevent long-term damage to the body.

Diagnosing Diabetes

The *fasting plasma glucose test* is the preferred test for diagnosing type 1 or type 2 diabetes. It is most reliable when done in the morning. However, a diagnosis of diabetes can be made after positive results on any one of the following three tests, with confirmation from a second positive test on a different day.

* ❖ A plasma glucose value of 126 mg/dL or higher after a person has fasted for eight hours
* ❖ An oral glucose tolerance test (OGTT) plasma glucose value of 200 mg/dL or higher in a blood sample taken two hours after a person has consumed a drink containing 75 grams of glucose dissolved in water. This test, taken in a laboratory or the doctor's office, measures plasma glucose at timed intervals over a three-hour period.
* ❖ A random (taken any time of day) plasma glucose value of 200 mg/dL or higher, along with the presence of diabetes symptoms

Gestational diabetes is diagnosed based on plasma glucose values measured during the OGTT. Glucose levels are normally lower during pregnancy, so the threshold values for diagnosis of diabetes in pregnancy are lower. If a woman has two plasma glucose values meeting or exceeding any of the following numbers, she has gestational diabetes: a fasting plasma glucose level of 95 mg/dL, a one-hour level of 180 mg/dL, a two-hour level of 155 mg/dL, or a three-hour level of 140 mg/dL. Let's take a closer look at the tests used for diagnosing diabetes.

Fasting Plasma Glucose (FPG) Test

A fasting plasma glucose test (FPG) measures your blood glucose after you have gone at least eight hours without eating. This test

TABLE 1.1 **Fasting Plasma Glucose Test (FPGT)**	
Plasma Glucose Result (mg/dL)	**Diagnosis**
99 and below	Normal
100 to 125	Prediabetes (impaired fasting glucose)
126 and above	Diabetes*

*Confirmed by repeating the test on a different day.

is used to detect diabetes or prediabetes. The FPG is the preferred test for diagnosing diabetes and is most reliable when done in the morning. (Results and their meaning are shown in Table 1.1.) If your fasting glucose level is 100 to 125 mg/dL, you have a form of prediabetes called *impaired fasting glucose* (*IFG*), meaning that you are more likely to develop type 2 diabetes but do not have it yet. A level of 126 mg/dL or higher, confirmed by repeating the test on another day, means that you have diabetes.

Oral Glucose Tolerance Test (OGTT)

An OGTT measures your blood glucose after you have gone at least eight hours without eating and two hours after you drink a glucose-containing beverage. This test can be used to diagnose diabetes or prediabetes. Research has shown that the OGTT is more sensitive than the FPG test for diagnosing prediabetes, but it is less convenient to administer. The OGTT requires you to fast for at least eight hours before the test; and then your plasma glucose is measured immediately before and two hours after you drink a liquid containing 75 grams of glucose dissolved in water. Results and what they mean are shown in Table 1.2. If your blood glucose level is between 140 and 199 mg/dL two hours after drinking the liquid, you have a form of prediabetes called *impaired glucose tolerance* (*IGT*), meaning that you are more likely

TABLE 1.2 Oral Glucose Tolerance Test (OGTT)

Two-Hour Plasma Glucose Result (mg/dL)	Diagnosis
139 and below	Normal
140 to 199	Prediabetes (impaired glucose tolerance)
200 and above	Diabetes*

*Confirmed by repeating the test on a different day.

to develop type 2 diabetes but do not have it yet. A two-hour glucose level of 200 mg/dL or higher, confirmed by repeating the test on another day, means that you have diabetes.

Gestational diabetes is also diagnosed based on plasma glucose values measured during the OGTT. Blood glucose levels are checked four times during the test. If your blood glucose levels are above normal at least twice during the test, you have gestational diabetes. Table 1.3 shows the above-normal results for the OGTT for gestational diabetes.

For additional information about the diagnosis and treatment of gestational diabetes, call the National Diabetes Information Clearinghouse (NDIC) at 1-800-860-8747.

TABLE 1.3 Results for the OGTT for Gestational Diabetes

When	Plasma Glucose Result (mg/dL)
Fasting	95 or higher
At 1 hour	180 or higher
At 2 hours	155 or higher
At 3 hours	140 or higher

Note: Some laboratories use other numbers for this test.

Random Plasma Glucose Test

In a random plasma glucose test, your doctor checks your blood glucose without regard to when you ate your last meal. This test, along with an assessment of symptoms, is used to diagnose diabetes but not prediabetes. A random blood glucose level of 200 mg/dL or higher, plus presence of the following symptoms, may indicate that you have diabetes:

* Increased urination
* Increased thirst
* Unexplained weight gain

Other symptoms include fatigue, blurred vision, increased hunger, and sores that do not heal. Your doctor will check your blood glucose level on another day using the FPG or the OGTT to confirm the diagnosis.

Highs and Lows of Diabetes: Hyperglycemia and Hypoglycemia

If your blood glucose stays higher than 180, it may be too high—a condition called *hyperglycemia*. It means you don't have enough insulin in your body. High blood glucose can happen if you miss taking your diabetes medicine, eat too much, or don't get enough exercise. Sometimes, the medications you take for other problems cause high blood glucose. Be sure to tell your doctor about other medications that you take, including nutritional or herbal supplements.

Having an infection or being sick or under stress can also make your blood glucose too high. That's why it's very important to check your blood glucose and keep taking your insulin or diabetes pills when you're sick. If you're very thirsty and tired, have blurry vision, and have to go to the bathroom often, your blood glucose may be too high. Very high blood glucose may also make you feel sick to your stomach. Finally, if your blood glucose is high much of the time or if you have symptoms of high blood glucose, call your doctor. You may need a change in your insulin, diabetes pills, or in your meal plan.

Hypoglycemia happens when your blood glucose drops too low. It can come on fast and is caused by taking too much of your diabetes medication, missing or delaying a meal, exercising more than usual, or drinking too much alcohol. Sometimes, medications you take for other health problems can cause blood glucose to drop. Hypoglycemia can make you feel weak, confused, irritable, hungry, or tired. You may sweat a lot or get a headache. You may feel shaky. If your blood glucose drops lower, you could pass out or have a seizure. If you have any of these symptoms, check your blood glucose. If the level is 70 or lower, have one of the following right away:

✢ Two or three glucose tablets
✢ ½ cup (4 oz.) of any fruit juice
✢ A piece of fruit or a small box of raisins
✢ ½ cup (4 oz.) of a regular (not diet) soft drink
✢ Five or six pieces of hard candy
✢ One or two teaspoons of sugar or honey

After fifteen minutes, check your blood glucose again to make sure that it's no longer too low. Once your blood glucose is stable, if it will be at least an hour before your next meal, have a snack.

If you take insulin or a diabetes pill that can cause hypoglycemia, always carry food for emergencies. It's also a good idea to wear a medical identification bracelet or necklace. Tell your doctor if you have hypoglycemia often—especially at the same time of the day or night several times in a row—or if you've passed out from hypoglycemia. In addition, ask your doctor about *glucagon*, a medicine given as an injection with a syringe that quickly raises blood glucose. If you pass out from hypoglycemia, someone should call 911 and give you a glucagon shot. You can keep a glucagon kit at home and also at a few other places where you go often. Show your family, friends, and coworkers how to give you an injection if you pass out because of hypoglycemia.

Even if you don't use insulin, you should still tell your doctor about other medicines you are taking or if you have hypoglycemia often—especially at the same time of the day or night several times in a row. In addition, some diabetes pills other than insulin can cause hypoglycemia, so be sure to ask your doctor whether your pills can cause this condition.

You can prevent hypoglycemia by eating regular meals, taking your diabetes medication, and checking your blood glucose often. Checking will tell you whether your glucose level is going down. You can then take steps, like eating some fruit, crackers, or other snacks, to raise your blood glucose. When you have hypoglycemia, have a snack to bring your blood glucose back to normal.

Complications of Diabetes

Diabetes is a serious disease. Take good care of your diabetes so you will feel better and avoid the health problems diabetes can cause such as:

* Heart disease and stroke
* Eye disease that can lead to vision problems or even going blind
* Gum disease and loss of teeth
* Kidney problems
* Nerve damage that can cause your hands and feet to feel numb, which can lead to loss of a foot or a leg

When your diabetes is under control, you are more likely to feel better and be less tired and thirsty and urinate less often. You will heal better and have fewer gum, skin, or bladder infections and will be less likely to have blurry vision or numb hands or feet.

Heart Disease and Diabetes

Cardiovascular disease (CVD) is a major complication and the leading cause of premature death among people with diabetes. At least 65 percent of people with diabetes die from heart disease or stroke. Adults with diabetes are two to four times more likely to have heart disease or suffer a stroke than people without it. Middle-aged people with type 2 diabetes have the same high risk for heart attack as people without diabetes who already have had a heart attack.

Relatively small improvements in blood glucose (sugar), lipids, and blood pressure values result in decreased risk for diabetes complications. People with type 2 diabetes have high rates of *hypertension* (chronically elevated high blood pressure), *dyslipidemia*, and obesity, major reasons for their two-to-four-fold higher rates of CVD.

Let's look at the statistics:

- ❖ Ninety-seven percent of adults with type 2 diabetes have one or more lipid abnormalities and about 70 percent of people with diabetes also have high blood pressure.
- ❖ Sticky blood platelets contribute to clotting problems and poor blood flow in people with diabetes.
- ❖ Smoking doubles the risk for CVD in people with diabetes.
- ❖ Deaths from heart disease in women with diabetes have *increased* 23 percent over the past thirty years compared to a 27 percent *decrease* in women without diabetes.
- ❖ Heart attacks occur at an earlier age in people with diabetes.

❖ Deaths from heart disease in men with diabetes have decreased by only 13 percent compared to a 36 percent decrease in men without diabetes.

❖ People with diabetes are more likely to die from a heart attack and are more likely than those without diabetes to have a second event.

The biggest problem for people with diabetes is heart and blood vessel disease. Heart and blood vessel disease can lead to heart attacks and strokes. It also causes poor blood flow (circulation) in the legs and feet. To check for heart and blood vessel disease, your health-care team will do some tests. At least once a year, have a blood test to see how much cholesterol is in your blood. Your health-care provider should take your blood pressure at every visit. He or she may also check the circulation in your legs, feet, and neck. The best way to prevent heart and blood vessel disease is to take good care of yourself and your diabetes by doing the following:

❖ Eat foods that are low in fat and salt.
❖ Keep your blood glucose on track. Know your A1C. The target for most people is under 7.
❖ If you smoke, quit.
❖ Exercise regularly.
❖ Lose weight if you need to.
❖ Ask your health-care team whether you should take an aspirin every day.
❖ Keep your blood pressure on track. The target for most people is lower than 130/80. If needed, take medicine to control your blood pressure.

Blood pressure levels tell how much your blood is pushing against the walls of your blood vessels. Your pressure is given as two numbers. The first is the pressure as your heart beats and the second is the pressure as your heart relaxes. If your blood pressure is higher than your target, talk with your health-care team about changing your meal plan, adding exercise, losing weight, or taking medicine.

In addition, keep your cholesterol level on track. Cholesterol is a waxlike substance found in the body, and it appears in different forms. The target for LDL ("bad") cholesterol for most people is lower than 100. If needed, take medicine to control your blood fat levels. If your LDL cholesterol is 100 or higher, you are at increased risk of heart disease and may need treatment. A high level of total cholesterol also means a greater risk of heart disease.

But HDL ("good") cholesterol protects you from heart disease, so the higher it is, the better. It's best to keep triglyceride (a type of fat) levels under 150. All of these target numbers are important for preventing heart disease.

Vision and Diabetes

Have your eyes checked once a year. You could have eye problems that you haven't noticed yet and it is important to catch them early when they can be treated. Treating eye problems early can help prevent blindness. High blood glucose can make the blood vessels in the eyes bleed, which can lead to blindness. You can help prevent eye damage by keeping your blood glucose as close to normal as possible. If your eyes are already damaged, an eye doctor may be able to save your sight with laser treatments or surgery.

The best way to prevent eye disease is to have a yearly eye exam. The eye doctor puts drops in your eyes to make your pupils get bigger (dilate). When the pupils are big, the doctor can see into the back of the eye. This is called a *dilated eye exam*, and it doesn't hurt. If you've never had this kind of eye exam before, you should have one now, even if you haven't had any trouble with your eyes. Be sure to tell your eye doctor that you have diabetes.

Here are some additional tips for taking care of your eyes:

❖ If you have type 1 diabetes, have your eyes examined when you have had it for five years and then every year after that first exam. (Children should have an eye exam in their early teens.)
❖ If you have type 2 diabetes, have an eye exam every year.
❖ If you are a woman planning to have a baby, have an eye exam before becoming pregnant.
❖ If you smoke, quit.
❖ Keep your blood glucose and blood pressure as close to normal as possible.

Tell your eye doctor right away if you have any problems such as blurry vision or seeing dark spots, flashing lights, or rings around lights.

Diabetes and Your Kidneys

Your kidneys help clean waste products from your blood. They also work to keep the right balance of salt and fluid in your body. Too much glucose in your blood is very hard on your kidneys. After a number of years, uncontrolled high blood glucose brings about increased stress on the kidneys by causing them to filter excess protein and glucose. Over time, this can lead to the kidneys deteriorating, a condition that eventually leads to kidney failure. If your kidneys stop working, you'll need dialysis (using a machine or special fluids to clean your blood) or a kidney transplant.

Have a urine test once a year for signs of kidney damage. The test measures how much protein is in your urine. A type of blood pressure medicine called an *ACE inhibitor* can help prevent kidney damage. Ask your doctor whether this medicine could help you. To help prevent kidney problems:

❖ Keep your blood glucose and blood pressure as close to normal as possible.

❖ Take your medicine if you have high blood pressure.

❖ Ask your doctor or your dietitian whether you should eat less meat, cheese, milk, fish, or fewer eggs.

❖ See your doctor right away if you get a bladder or kidney infection. Signs of bladder or kidney infections are cloudy or bloody urine, pain or burning when you urinate, and having to urinate often or in a hurry. Back pain, chills, and fever are also signs of kidney infection.

❖ Quit smoking.

Diabetes and Your Nerves

Over time, high blood glucose can harm the nerves in your body. Nerve damage can cause you to lose the feeling in your feet or to have painful, burning feet. It can also cause pain in your legs, arms, or hands or cause problems with eating, going to the bathroom, or having sex. Nerve damage can happen slowly and you may not even realize you have problems. Your doctor should check your nerves at least once a year. Part of this exam should include tests to check your sense of feeling and the pulse in your feet. Tell the doctor about any problems with your feet, legs, hands, or arms. Also, let the doctor know if you are having trouble eating, going to the bathroom, or having sex or if you feel dizzy sometimes.

Nerve damage to the feet can lead to amputations. You may not feel pain from injuries or sore spots on your feet, but if you have poor circulation because of blood vessel problems in your legs, the sores on your feet can't heal and might become infected. If the infection isn't treated, it could lead to amputation. Ask your doctor whether you already have nerve damage in your feet. If you do, it is especially important to take good care of them. To help prevent complications from nerve damage, check your feet every day.

Here are some additional ways to take care of your nerves:

* Keep your blood glucose and blood pressure as close to normal as possible.
* Limit the amount of alcohol you drink.
* Check your feet every day.
* If you smoke, quit.

Foot Care Tips. Keep your blood glucose in your target range and take care of your feet to help protect them. In addition, you can do a lot to prevent problems with your feet. Take a look at the following tips.

* **Check your bare feet every day.** Look for cuts, sores, bumps, or red spots. Use a mirror or ask a family member for help if you have trouble seeing the bottoms of your feet.

* **Wash your feet in warm—not hot—water every day, but don't soak them.** Use mild soap. Dry your feet with a soft towel, and dry carefully between your toes.

* **After washing your feet, cover them with lotion before putting your shoes and socks on.** Don't put lotion or cream between your toes.

* **File your toenails straight across with an emery board.** Don't leave sharp edges that could cut the next toe.

* **Don't try to cut calluses or corns off with a razor blade or knife, and don't use wart removers on your feet.** If you have warts or painful corns or calluses, see a podiatrist, a doctor who treats foot problems.

* **Wear thick, soft socks.** Don't wear mended socks or stockings with holes or seams that might rub against your feet.

* **Check your shoes before you put them on.** You want to be sure they have no sharp edges or objects in them.

* **Wear shoes that fit well and let your toes move.** Break new shoes in slowly. Don't wear flip-flops, shoes with pointed toes, or plastic shoes. Never go barefoot.

❖ **Wear socks if your feet get cold at night.** Don't use heating pads or hot water bottles on your feet.

❖ **Have your doctor check your feet at every visit.** Take your shoes and socks off when you go into the examining room. This will remind the doctor to check your feet.

❖ **See a podiatrist for help if you can't take care of your feet yourself.**

Diabetes and Your Gums and Teeth

Diabetes can lead to infections in your gums and the bones that hold your teeth in place. Like all infections, gum infections can cause blood glucose to rise. Without treatment, teeth may become loose and fall out.

To help prevent damage to your gums and teeth look at the following tips:

❖ See your dentist twice a year. Tell your dentist that you
    have diabetes.
❖ Brush and floss your teeth at least twice a day.
❖ If you smoke, quit.
❖ Keep your blood glucose as close to normal as possible.

To best prevent gum disease, keep your blood glucose in your target range, brush and floss your teeth every day, and have regular dental checkups.

Now that you have a basic understanding of the symptoms and complications of diabetes, we'll look more closely at the dietary factors that can have an impact on your health.

Taking Control of Diabetes

WHAT YOU EAT has a big impact on your health. In this chapter, we'll discuss how controlling portion sizes, exercising, and achieving a healthy weight can help you to stabilize your diabetes and prevent complications like cardiovascular disease and metabolic syndrome, which we'll look at in detail in Chapter 3.

Weighing In: Striving for a Healthy Weight

Your weight affects your health in many ways. Being overweight can keep your body from making and using insulin properly as well as cause high blood pressure. The Diabetes Prevention Program (DPP) showed that losing even a few pounds can help reduce your risk of developing type 2 diabetes because your body learns to use insulin more effectively. In the DPP, people who lost between 5 and 7 percent of their body weight significantly reduced their risk of type 2 diabetes. For example, if you weigh two hundred pounds, losing only ten pounds could make a difference. If you have diabetes, losing weight will help to prevent complications.

Body mass index, or *BMI*, is a measure of body weight relative to height. You can use BMI to see whether you are underweight, normal weight, overweight, or obese. Use the body mass index table (Table 2.1) to find your BMI.

TABLE 2.1 Estimating Your BMI

Height	\ Weight (in Pounds)															
	100	**110**	**120**	**130**	**140**	**150**	**160**	**170**	**180**	**190**	**200**	**210**	**220**	**230**	**240**	**250**
5′	20	21	23	25	27	29	31	33	35	37	39	41	43	45	47	49
5′1″	19	21	23	25	26	28	30	32	34	36	38	40	42	43	45	47
5′2″	18	20	22	24	26	27	29	31	33	35	37	38	40	42	44	46
5′3″	18	19	21	23	25	27	28	30	32	34	35	37	39	41	43	44
5′4″	17	19	21	22	24	26	27	29	31	33	34	36	38	39	41	43
5′5″	17	18	20	22	23	25	27	28	30	32	33	35	37	38	40	42
5′6″	16	18	19	21	23	24	26	27	29	31	32	34	36	37	39	40
5′7″	16	17	19	20	22	23	25	27	28	30	31	33	34	36	38	39
5′8″	15	17	18	20	21	23	24	26	27	29	30	32	33	35	36	38
5′9″	15	16	18	19	21	22	24	25	27	28	30	31	32	34	35	37
5′10″	14	16	17	19	20	22	23	24	26	27	29	30	32	33	34	36
5′11″	14	15	17	18	20	21	22	24	25	26	28	29	31	32	33	35
6′	14	15	16	18	19	20	22	23	24	26	27	28	30	31	33	34
6′1″	13	15	16	17	18	20	21	22	24	25	26	28	29	30	32	33
6′2″	13	14	15	17	18	19	21	22	23	24	26	27	28	30	31	32
6′3″	12	14	15	16	17	19	20	21	22	24	25	26	27	29	30	31
6′4″	12	13	15	16	17	18	19	21	22	23	24	26	27	28	29	30

1. Find your height in the left-hand column.
2. Move across in the same row to the number closest to your weight.
3. The number in that column is your BMI. Check your BMI and talk with your doctor to help you achieve a healthy weight.

Get Moving! How Exercise Helps

Regular exercise tackles several risk factors at once. It helps you lose weight, keeps your cholesterol and blood pressure under control, and helps your body use blood sugar for energy. The Diabetes Prevention Program (DPP) showed that people who were physically active for thirty minutes a day five days a week reduced their risk of type 2 diabetes by 58 percent. Exercise also has been found to prevent cardiac dysfunction in diabetes patients.

If you are not currently active, start slowly—first talk with your doctor about which kinds of exercise would be safe for you. Make a plan to increase your activity level toward the goal of being active for at least thirty minutes a day most days of the week.

Choose activities you enjoy. Here are some additional ways to work extra activity into your daily routine:

* Take the stairs rather than an elevator or escalator.
* Park at the far end of the lot and walk.
* Get off the bus a few stops early and walk the rest of the way.
* Whenever you can, walk or bicycle instead of drive.

Diet and Your Diabetes

Take a hard look at the serving sizes of the foods you eat. Reduce serving sizes of meat, desserts, and foods high in fat. Increase your daily intake of fruits and vegetables. (In Chapter 6, we will discuss in depth the foods that help to stabilize blood sugar.)

Limit your total fat to 25 to 30 percent of your calories. For example, if you consume 2,000 calories a day, try to eat no more than 56 to 65 grams of fat each day. Your doctor or a dietitian can help you figure out how much daily fat you need. Be sure to read food labels for fat content, too. (In Chapter 8, we give you some smart shopping tips and healthy choices when dining out).

If you are overweight, you need to cut back on the number of calories you consume each day. People who participated in the DPP lifestyle modification group lowered their daily calorie total by an average of about 450 calories. Your doctor or dietitian can help you with a daily calorie-level meal plan that emphasizes weight loss. (We provide you with simple meal plans for a 1,200 calorie and a 1,600 calorie weight-loss plan in addition to a 2,000 calorie plan in Chapter 9, as well as quick and delicious recipes in Chapter 10.)

Keep a food and exercise log. Write down what you eat, how much you exercise you get, and anything else that helps keep you on track. Research shows that successful weight losers consistently monitor what they eat and how often they exercise. When you meet your goal, reward yourself with a nonfood item or activity, such as watching a movie, going out with friends, or buying yourself something personal—like a size smaller dress or pants.

Portion Distortion: An Eye on Size

"Portion distortion" is everywhere, however. Most Americans don't realize that it leads to super-sized health problems. The portion size at most fast-food restaurants has increased, and studies show that people will eat more when presented with a bigger portion. Worse yet, Americans underestimate the number of calories they consume by 25 to 50 percent. Fifty excess calories a day over a ten-year period will increase your weight by fifty pounds! Or, cut 100 calories a day, and you will drop seven pounds in a year. However, food isn't the only culprit. Soda guzzling can tack on calories and pounds as well.

Simple kitchen tools, such as measuring cups and spoons or a food scale, can help you to ensure your food servings are the right size. Weigh and measure your foods to make sure you eat the right amounts, which will help you to control your weight and manage your diabetes.

❖ **For dry foods, like cereal, pasta, or rice.** Measure and pour it into a bowl or plate. The next time you eat that food, use the same bowl or plate and fill it to the same level.

❖ **For beverages.** Measure one cup and pour it into a glass. See how high it fills the glass. Always drink beverages, other than water, from that sized glass.

❖ **For meat.** Remember that meat weighs more prior to cooking. For example, four ounces of raw meat will weigh about three ounces after cooking. For meat with a bone—such as a pork chop or chicken leg—cook five ounces raw to get three ounces cooked. In addition, one serving of meat or meat substitute is about the size and thickness of a deck of cards.

In addition, these tips will help you choose the right serving sizes:

❖ A small fist is equal to about one-half cup of fruit, vegetables, or starches like rice.
❖ A small fist is equal to one small piece of fresh fruit.
❖ A thumb is equal to about one ounce of meat or cheese.
❖ The tip of a thumb is equal to about one teaspoon.

In the next chapter, we'll discuss insulin resistance and metabolic syndrome, their relationship with diabetes and heart disease, and the dietary strategies to keep healthy.

The Link: Insulin Resistance, Diabetes, and Metabolic Syndrome

LIKE A THIEF in the night, insulin resistance is a silent condition that robs you of your health by increasing the chances of developing diabetes and heart disease. With this condition, your muscle, fat, and liver cells do not use insulin properly, and the pancreas tries to keep up with the demand for insulin by producing more. Eventually, the pancreas cannot keep up with the body's need for insulin, and excess glucose builds up in the bloodstream. Think of your pancreas as a garden hose (producing insulin), your cells as a bucket (catching insulin), and the insulin as water. With insulin resistance, the spigot is not turned off in time, the bucket overflows and spills into your proverbial bloodstream, causing a plethora of problems that rob you of your health.

People with blood glucose levels that are higher than normal but not yet in the diabetic range have *prediabetes*. Doctors sometimes call this condition *impaired fasting glucose* (*IFG*) or *impaired glucose tolerance* (*IGT*), depending on the test used to diagnose it. In a cross section of U.S. adults aged forty to seventy-four tested during the period from 1988 to 1994, 33.8 percent had IFG, 15.4 percent had IGT, and 40.1 percent had prediabetes (IGT or IFG or both). Applying these percentages to the U.S. population in the year 2000, about thirty-five million adults aged forty to seventy-four would have IFG, sixteen million would have IGT, and forty-one million would have prediabetes.

Prediabetes greatly increases your risk of developing type 2 diabetes, formerly called adult-onset diabetes or non-insulin-dependent diabetes (NIDDM). Studies have shown that most people with prediabetes go on to develop type 2 diabetes within ten years, unless they lose 5 to 7 percent of their body weight—about ten to fifteen pounds for someone who weighs two hundred pounds—by making modest changes in their diet and level of physical activity. People with prediabetes also have a higher risk of heart disease.

Metabolic Syndrome: The Deadly Quartet

The National Cholesterol Education Program has found four health bandits on the loose, collectively defined as *metabolic syndrome*, also known as *insulin resistance syndrome*. The presence of any three of the four of the "deadly quartet" indicates foul play (the diagnosis). Let's take a look at the lineup.

* Excess weight around the waist (waist measurement of more than forty inches for men and more than thirty-five inches for women)
* High levels of triglycerides (150 mg/dL or higher)
* Low levels of HDL, or "good" cholesterol (below 40 mg/dL for men and below 50 mg/dL for women)
* High blood pressure (130/85 mm Hg higher)
* High fasting blood glucose levels (110 mg/dL or higher)

Risk Factors for Metabolic Syndrome

Having one of the bandits lingering means it's likely the others are on their way. Therefore, it's important that anyone forty-five years or older should consider getting tested for diabetes, especially if you are overweight. In addition, consider getting tested if you are younger than forty-five, overweight, and have one or more of the following risk factors:

* Family history of diabetes
* Low HDL cholesterol and high triglycerides
* High blood pressure
* History of gestational diabetes (diabetes during pregnancy) or gave birth to a baby weighing more than nine pounds
* Minority group background (African American, American Indian, Hispanic American/Latino, or Asian American/ Pacific Islander)

Tests for Metabolic Syndrome

Diabetes and prediabetes can be detected with one of these four tests.

* **Blood glucose.** High blood glucose may be a sign that your body does not have enough insulin or does not use it well. However, a fasting measurement or oral glucose tolerance test gives more precise information.
* **Insulin.** An insulin measurement helps determine whether a high blood glucose reading is the result of insufficient insulin or poor use of insulin.
* **Fasting glucose.** Your blood glucose level should be lower after several hours without eating. After an overnight fast, the normal level is below 100 mg/dL. If it is in the 100 to 125

mg/dL range, you have impaired fasting glucose or prediabetes. A result of 126 or higher, if confirmed on a repeat test, indicates diabetes.

✿ **Glucose tolerance.** Your blood glucose level will be higher after drinking a sugar solution, but it should still be below 140 mg/dL two hours after the drink. If it is higher than normal (in the 140 to 199 mg/dL range) two hours after drinking the solution, you have IGT or prediabetes, which is another strong indication that your body has trouble using glucose. A level of 200 or higher, if confirmed, means diabetes is already present.

Preventing and Reversing Metabolic Syndrome

Physical inactivity and excess weight are open invitations for the deadly quartet. Losing weight and getting more exercise can send these bandits packing—helping to reduce or prevent the complications associated with metabolic syndrome. In 2001, the National Institutes of Health completed the DPP, a clinical trial designed to find the most effective ways of preventing type 2 diabetes in overweight people with prediabetes. The researchers found that lifestyle changes reduced the risk of diabetes by 58 percent. Also, many people with prediabetes returned to normal blood glucose levels.

Physical activity helps your muscle cells use blood glucose because they need it for energy. Exercise makes those cells more sensitive to insulin, allowing the insulin to be properly utilized, preventing the "overflow" in the bucket example we referred to earlier. The DPP confirmed that people who increase activities such as walking briskly or riding a bike for thirty minutes, five times a week, have a far smaller risk of developing diabetes than people who do not exercise regularly.

The DPP also reinforced the importance of following a low-calorie, low-fat diet, which can provide two benefits. If you are overweight, one benefit is that limiting your calorie and fat intake can help you lose weight. DPP participants who lost weight were far less likely to develop diabetes than others in the study who remained at an unhealthy weight. Increasing your activity and eating a healthy diet can also improve your blood pressure and cholesterol levels as well as provide many other health benefits.

Smoking, in addition to increasing your risk of cancer and cardiovascular disease, also contributes to insulin resistance.

Scientists have established some numbers to help people set goals that will reduce their risk of developing glucose metabolism problems.

❖ **Weight.** Body mass index (BMI) is a measure used to evaluate body weight relative to height. You can use BMI (from Chapter 2) to find out whether you are underweight, normal weight, overweight, or obese.

❖ **Blood pressure.** Blood pressure is expressed as two numbers that represent pressure in your blood vessels when your heart is beating (systolic pressure) and when it is resting (diastolic pressure). The numbers are usually written with a slash—for example, 140/90, which is expressed as "140 over 90." For the general population, blood pressure below 130/85 is considered normal. However, people who have a blood pressure that is slightly elevated and who have no additional risk factors for heart disease may be advised to make lifestyle changes—that is, diet and exercise—rather than taking blood pressure medicines. People who have diabetes, however, should take whatever steps necessary, including lifestyle changes and medicine, to reach a blood pressure goal of below 130/80.

❖ **Cholesterol.** Your cholesterol levels are usually reported with three values: low density lipoprotein (LDL) cholesterol, high density lipoprotein (HDL) cholesterol, and total cholesterol. LDL cholesterol is sometimes called "bad" cholesterol, while HDL cholesterol is called "good" cholesterol. To lower your risk of cardiovascular problems if you have diabetes, you should try to keep your LDL cholesterol below 100 and your total cholesterol below 200.

The Role of Inflammation in Metabolic Syndrome

Adipocytes, or fat cells, are the proverbial revolvers of the deadly quartet. Never holstered and always firing, fat cells shoot out inflammatory factors called *cytokines*. Like wounding bullets, these cytokines (including tumor necrosis factor, interleukin, and C-reactive protein) get in the way of normal bodily functions and have negative effects on hormones. Because more fat cells are present, being overweight or obese is associated with a state of inflammation. In the past ten years, researchers have found these fat-cell produced cytokines are related to insulin resistance, type 2 diabetes, cardiovascular disease, and metabolic syndrome.

One especially dangerous cytokine, C-reactive protein (CRP), is so powerful that its presence predicts the risk of cardiovascular disease. Because blood sugar stimulates the release of cytokines, decreasing fasting glucose is an important factor in preventing heart-harming events. The higher the blood sugar level, the more C-reactive protein produced in the body and the greater the risk of cardiovascular complications.

This tiny factor is not to be reckoned with. In fact, it's even on the American Heart Association's "most wanted" list. A recent report published by the American Heart Association/Centers for Disease Control and Prevention (AHA/CDC) duo indicates that CRP measurements may provide important information for assessing heart disease beyond that which may be obtained from established risk factors. Talk with your doctor about checking your levels of CRP, and we'll show you how to deflate this inflamed predator and send the deadly quartet packing with the foods you eat in the next section.

Reducing Inflammation Through Diet

Research shows that diet can act as a stealthy militia in guarding your health and disarming the deadly quartet. Antioxidant phytonutrients and fiber found in plant foods step up to the call of duty to decrease inflammation and defuse inflammatory weaponry, while certain fats and carbs only add to the health-harming arsenal. Let's take a look at the research.

Fiber, Grains, and Glycemic Load. A number of studies have found a relation between high-fiber, whole-grain, and low-glycemic-index foods (which we'll discuss in detail in Chapter 4) and reduced signs of inflammation.

A study of 732 healthy women from the Nurses' Health Study were evaluated using a food frequency questionnaire, a tool that analyzes what foods they ate and how often they ate them. The study compared women consuming a "prudent" pattern diet—higher intakes of fruit, vegetables, legumes, fish, poultry, and whole grains—with those consuming a Western pattern diet, characterized by higher intakes of red and processed meats, sweets, desserts, french fries, and refined grains. The prudent pattern was inversely associated with levels of CRP, whereas the Western pattern showed a positive relation with CRP, interleukin 6, and other factors of inflammation.

Similarly, the National Health and Nutrition Examination Survey (NHANES 99-00) found that fiber intake was inversely associated with CRP levels. We have many recipes in Chapter 10 that are loaded with fiber, and we point those out to you in that chapter. Similarly, the Health Eating Index (HEI), a measure of diet quality according to the Dietary Guidelines for Americans, was examined for its effect on CRP. Among the components measured, researchers concluded that whole-grain consumption may reduce inflammation, as whole-grain consumption was inversely associated with CRP levels.

Studies on metabolism have shown that a high intake of rapidly digested and absorbed carbohydrates can lead to an insulin resistance. These quickly digested carbohydrates—ranking high on a scale called the *glycemic index*—deliver sugar to the bloodstream, causing insulin levels to spike. The glycemic index was created to quantify and rank the body's response to different carbohydrate-containing foods.

Fruits, Vegetables and Their Anti-Inflammatory Action. Partly because of their diverse mix of phytonutrients, veggie vigilantes (and fruits, too) help to reduce those inflammatory factors that increase the risk for cardiovascular disease.

A recent study conducted at the Jean Mayer U.S. Department of Agriculture, Human Nutrition Research Center on Aging at Tufts examined the relationship between CRP, homocysteine (Hcy), and the intake of fruits and vegetables. The study found that frequent consumption of fruits and vegetables is associated with lower concentrations of both CRP and Hcy. Because these compounds are known instigators of cardiovascular disease, eating more fruits and vegetables may be an effective strategy to protect the heart.

One group of phytonutrients in particular, *flavonoids*, have been studied for their anti-inflammatory action. Found in high concentrations in cocoa, red wine, and tea, most studies show an inverse association between flavonoid consumption and the risk of cardiovascular disease, as well as diabetes.

Researchers believe that as a class, flavonoids halt the oxidation of LDL cholesterol, reduce the potential for a dangerous clot, improve the function of red blood cells, and alter the pathways that lead to inflammation. We will describe flavonoids and other diabetes-beating phytonutrients in Chapter 5.

The Homocysteine and Heart Disease Link. Homocysteine, an ally of the deadly quartet and an amino acid found normally in the body, also increases a person's risk of heart disease, stroke, and peripheral vascular disease (a reduced blood flow to the hands and feet).

Numerous studies, including the Physicians' Health Study, the Tromso Study from Norway, the Framingham Heart Study, and a meta-analysis of nearly forty studies have found that people with elevated levels of Hcy in their blood are at an increased risk of heart disease.

Scientists have several theories. First, a high level of Hcy may be involved with the process called *atherosclerosis*, the gradual buildup of fatty substances in arteries. Homocysteine also may make blood more likely to clot by increasing the stickiness of blood platelets. Clots can block blood flow, causing a heart attack or stroke. Increased Hcy may affect other substances involved in clotting too. Finally, higher Hcy levels may make blood vessels less flexible—and so less able to widen to increase blood flow.

However the veggie vigilantes mentioned earlier can disarm this ally of the deadly quartet thanks to foods rich in folate, vitamin B_6, and vitamin B_{12}. These B vitamins actually help to reduce levels of heart-harming homocysteine. Take a look at some of the health sources that are heroes against homocysteine.

❖ **Sources of folate (per serving).** Black-eyed peas (105 mcg or 25% DV), cooked spinach (100 mcg or 25% DV), great northern beans (90 mcg or 20% DV), asparagus (85 mcg or 20% DV), wheat germ (40 mcg or 10% DV), orange juice (35 mcg or 10% DV), peas (50 mcg or 15% DV), cooked broccoli (45 mcg or 15% DV), avocado (45 mcg or 10% DV), and peanuts (40 mcg or 10% DV).

❖ **Sources of vitamin B_6 (per serving).** Potatoes (0.7 mg or 35% DV), garbanzo beans (0.57 or 30% DV), chicken breast (0.52 mg or 25% DV), oatmeal (0.42 mg or 20% DV), trout (0.29 mg or 15% DV), sunflower seeds (0.23 mg or 10% DV), avocado (0.20 mg or 10% DV), tuna (0.18mg or 10% DV), and cooked spinach (0.14 mg or 8% DV).

✤ **Sources of vitamin B$_{12}$ (per serving).** Clams (84.1 mg or 1,400% DV), trout (5.4 mg or 90% DV), salmon (4.9 mg or 80% DV), yogurt (1.4 mg or 25% DV) tuna (1 mg or 15% DV), milk (0.9 mg or 15% DV).

Now that you have an understanding of the factors and ways to control metabolic syndrome, in the next chapter we'll discuss the fats and carbohydrates that pick sides in the battle against diabetes and heart disease and how to spot your friends and foes.

Fats, Carbs, and Diabetes

MIXED MESSAGES ON FATS and carbohydrates have led many Americans down a road of degenerating health. First, we hear that fat is bad, and carbohydrates (or carbs) are good. Then, we are fed the notion that severely limiting carbs—and all the wonderfully nutritious foods they are found in—will help us lose weight. A healthy weight is a key factor in preventing diseases, including diabetes, however, these efforts have proven unsuccessful as an astounding 50 percent of Americans are overweight. The truth of the matter and common denominator among fats and carbs is that *there are good ones and there are bad ones.*

The *glycemic index (GI)*, a new system for classifying carbs, gives us greater insight to the "all carbs are bad" myth and helps us separate the wheat from the chaff (no pun intended). By measuring how fast and how far blood sugar rises after consuming a carb-rich food, we better understand the impact foods have on diabetes and our metabolism.

Although such a system does not exist for fats, numerous studies have proven the "friends" and "foes" of the fat world. Some fats increase insulin resistance, raise cholesterol, and make platelets sticky—raising the risk for a heart attack or stroke. Others allow the arteries to open up and increase levels of "good" cholesterol (HDL) and enhance insulin sensitivity.

When you eliminate good carbs and good fats, you also forgo the critical nutrients that help to balance blood sugar and protect the heart. Afraid of fat so you skip the olive oil, nuts, and avocados? You're missing out on minerals such as magnesium, good fats, plus antioxidants. Under the impression that all carbs are bad, so you minimize carbohydrates in your diet? There go the fiber and phytoestrogens that work together to keep blood sugar on an even keel.

Healing Gourmet makes it easy for you to follow the principles discovered by modern science to benefit diabetes. In this chapter, we will point out the good guys and bad guys of the fat and carb world and show how they relate to diabetes and its complications.

Bad Fats and Diabetes

Structurally, fats are simple molecules built around a series of carbon atoms (C) linked to each other in a chain. Dietary fats are composed of long chains containing twelve to twenty-two carbons. A small change in the structure of a dietary fat can make a big impact on your overall health. First, let's take a look at the fat foes and their effects on insulin.

The Fat Foe: Saturated Fat

Saturated fats are mainly animal fats. They are found in meat, seafood, whole milk dairy products (cheese, milk, and ice cream), poultry skin, and egg yolks. Some plant foods are also high in saturated fats, including coconut and coconut oil, palm oil, and palm kernel oil. With saturated fatty acids, each of the interior carbon atoms is bonded to two hydrogen atoms as well as two other carbons. All of the bonds available for hydrogen are filled or "saturated" with hydrogen, hence the name.

Saturated Fat and Diabetes. Saturated fat in the diet stifles the function of the insulin-secreting cells of the pancreas (beta cells), reducing sensitivity to insulin. This fat foe also increases triglyceride levels and has negative effects on the kidneys (previously discussed in Chapter 1). How does this happen? As we consume saturated fats, they are stored in cells as triglycerides, causing damage to those cells. As these compounds increase in our insulin-secreting cells, the damage accumulates and causes these important cells to die.

The Health Professionals Follow-Up Study examined the relationship between dietary fat and meat intake to the risk of type 2 diabetes. The study followed 42,504 male participants for twelve years and found total and saturated fat intake were associated with a higher risk of type 2 diabetes. The study also showed that frequently eating processed meats—such as lunchmeat, hot dogs, or bacon—may increase the risk for type 2 diabetes.

Similarly, the Women's Health Study examined the relationship between red meat consumption and risk of type 2 diabetes. Over an eight year eight month period, 37,309 female participants—age forty-five or older who were free of disease (including cancer, heart disease and type 2 diabetes)—were given food frequency questionnaires (a survey of the types and amounts of foods eaten). The study showed that eating red and processed meat significantly increased the risk for type 2 diabetes, emphasizing a higher risk for those who frequently ate processed meat, including bacon and hot dogs.

 Healing Tip

By limiting or avoiding red and processed meat and full-fat dairy, you can minimize your exposure to the beta-cell bully, saturated fat. Opt instead for plant-based fats, fish, low-fat dairy, and lean poultry—preferably organic or free range.

The Foe: Trans Fat

Trans fatty acids are fats produced through a process called *hydrogenation*, which adds a hydrogen to the fat molecule. Hydrogenation became popular because this type of oil doesn't spoil or become rancid as easily as regular oil and therefore has a longer shelf life. The more hydrogenated an oil is, the harder it will be at room temperature. For example, a spreadable tub of margarine is less hydrogenated and so has fewer trans fats than a stick of margarine. Most of the trans fats in the American diet are found in commercially prepared baked goods, margarines, snack foods, and processed foods, as well as commercially prepared fried foods, such as french fries and onion rings. A report from the Institute of Medicine concluded that there is no safe level of trans fats in the diet. This prompted the FDA to require that all Nutrition Facts food labels include trans fats by January 1, 2006. Check food labels for hydrogenated oils; the higher on the list they appear, the more trans fats there are in the product. We talk more about understanding the labeling on foods in Chapter 8.

Trans Fats and Diabetes. Irrefutably, eating foods containing trans fats increases the risk for heart disease because of the action of these villainous fats on cholesterol. They have also been fingered for their negative impact on blood sugar and insulin, playing an evil instigator in the development of diabetes.

The Nurses' Health Study evaluated 823 women for markers of inflammation and found that eating trans-fat-containing foods increases *C-reactive protein* (*CRP*), which, as discussed in Chapter 3, is an inflammatory factor most associated with heart disease and diabetes. A similar Harvard study evaluated the effects of trans fats on patients with heart disease. This study showed that trans fats in the diet are associated with heart disease and that reducing them is an important step in secondary prevention.

The FDA based the trans fats rule on recent studies that indicate that consumption of trans fatty acids contributes to increased LDL cholesterol levels, which increase the risk of coronary heart disease. Recent information from the American Heart Association indicates that heart disease causes about 500,000 deaths annually and is the number-one cause of death in the United States. Thus, the FDA is proposing to provide for information on trans fatty acids in nutrition labeling and nutrient content and health claims in response to its importance to public health. Table 4.1 illustrates the amounts of trans fats in common foods.

TABLE 4.1 Trans Fatty Acids in One Serving of Selected Foods

Food	Trans Fatty Acids Grams per Serving
Pound cake	4.3
Microwave popcorn (regular)	2.2
Margarine (stick)	1.8–3.5
An average snack cracker	1.8–2.5
Vegetable shortening	1.4–4.2
Vanilla wafers	1.3
Chocolate chip cookies	1.2–2.7
French fries (fast food)	0.7–3.6
Margarine (tub, regular)	0.4–1.6
Doughnuts	0.3–3.8
Salad dressings (regular)	0.06–1.1
White bread	0.06–0.7
Ready-to-eat breakfast cereals	0.05–0.5
Chocolate candies	0.04–2.8
Vegetable oils	0.01–0.06
An average snack chip	0–1.2

*Fatty acid data from USDA food composition data, 1995

Healing Tip

To reduce the inflammatory factors associated with chronic diseases, root out trans fat by looking for "partially hydrogenated oils" or "vegetable shortening" on food labels. Health-food stores offer trans fat–free shortenings and baked goods that are trans fat free.

Good Fats and Diabetes

Let's take a look at the health-promoting fats that benefit insulin function and help reduce inflammatory processes involved with diabetes, metabolic syndrome, and heart disease.

The Friend: Monounsaturated Fats (MUFAs)

Monounsaturated fats (MUFAs) are derived from various vegetable sources including olives, nuts, and avocados. The double bond allows the monounsaturated fatty acid chain to be a bit more fluid, making them liquid at room temperature.

Like their friendly cousins, the polyunsaturated fats (PUFAs), MUFAs are best known for their ability to decrease blood cholesterol levels if part of a healthful diet. They have also been found to contribute to glycemic control, helping to keep blood sugar stable. In addition, foods containing MUFAs also contain a spectrum of diabetes-beating and heart-helping phytonutrients such as phenols, beta-sitosterol, and lutein. In Chapter 6, we will discuss how compounds in foods team up to protect our health, a phenomenon called *synergy*.

Monounsaturated Fats and Diabetes. A recent study conducted at the University of Kuopio, Finland, examined the relationship between fatty acids in the blood and glucose metabolism. After a three-week, high-saturated-fat diet, thirty-one subjects with impaired glucose tolerance were put on a "mono" (primarily monounsaturated fats) or "poly" (primarily polyunsaturated fats) diet for eight weeks. The study found that those subjects with higher amounts of oleic acid—a monounsaturated fat from olive oil—and alpha-linolenic acid—an omega-3 fatty acid—had the most improvement in fasting plasma glucose.

Evidence from the Mediterranean diet also supports this research showing that consumption of MUFA-rich olive oil helps to reduce inflammatory processes and risk for heart disease.

 Kitchen Prescription

Stock your kitchen with nuts, olive oil, and avocados to get the benefits of health-promoting MUFAs. Trade in your chips and pretzels for a MUFA-rich snack mix including popcorn popped in canola oil and raw almonds.

The Friend: Polyunsaturated Fats (PUFAs)

The human body needs fatty acids and can make all but two of them: linolenic acid and linoleic acid. These fats must be supplied by the diet, hence the term "essential fatty acids." Used by the body to maintain cell membranes and make hormone-like substances that regulate blood pressure, clotting, immune response, insulin function, and blood lipids, the PUFA side of the fat family gets special treatment for its good behavior and positive impact on health.

Omega-3 fatty acids, also known as linolenic acid, are essential fatty acids (EFAs) that come from both plant and animal sources. Given linolenic acid, the body can make *eicosapentaenoic acid* (*EPA*) and *docosahexaenoic acid* (*DHA*), the two major fatty acids in fish. The greatest amounts of EPA and DHA are found in oily, dark-fleshed fish that live in deep, cold waters such as tuna, bluefish, and salmon. Alpha-linolenic acid is the other essential fatty acid and is found most abundantly in canola oil (11%) but also in flaxseed, walnuts, and soybeans—which contain a balance of omega-3 fats.

Omega-6 fatty acids, also known as linoleic acid, are much more common in the American diet and are found in soybean oil, safflower oil, sunflower oil, corn oil, wheat germ, and sesame. Researchers postulate that because omega-6 fatty acids are more readily available and consumed in Western countries, and that because our Paleolithic ancestors consumed a balance of omega-3 to omega-6 fatty acids, an imbalance could negatively influence inflammatory processes associated with diabetes and heart disease.

To get the maximum health benefits from the PUFAs, the ratio of omega-3 to omega-6 in our diet should be two to one. Let's take a look at each of the essentials and their role in diabetes.

Omega-3 Fats and Diabetes. In human studies, omega-3 fatty acids were shown to improve many of the negative effects of insulin resistance by lowering blood pressure and triacylglycerol concentrations that hamper the function of insulin-secreting cells. Additionally, studies have shown that this essential fatty acid may also have beneficial effects on some of the complications of diabetes (previously discussed in Chapter 1), helping to protect the blood vessels and kidneys. Most famous for their role in protecting the heart, omega-3s have been found to

* Reduce inflammation
* Decrease the risk for a blood clot
* Prevent irregular heartbeats
* Reduce cholesterol
* Help blood vessels to dilate, reducing blood pressure

Omega-6 and Diabetes. While omega-6 fatty acids are "good" fats, there is a dark side to these characters that has been created by modern technology. Most foods we consume are high in omega-6s, which, when they are left unbalanced by their anti-inflammatory counterpart (omega-3), can lead to health problems including cardiovascular disease, cancer, and inflammatory and autoimmune diseases.

Remember to strive for a good balance of omega-3 to omega-6, which can be achieved by consuming more whole foods and following some of our practical tips.

 Kitchen Prescription

To improve your ratio of omega-3 fatty acids to omega-6 fatty acids:

* Choose canola oil to cook.
* Select walnuts as a snack.
* Look for new food products with enhanced omega-3s, including eggs, breads, and cereals.
* Try flaxseed meal or hempseed meal as an addition to smoothies, cereals, and baked goods.
* Include cold-water fish (like salmon and tuna) in your diet.

The Dish on Fish and Mercury. Although there is no doubt that including fish in your diet will deliver protective essential fatty acids and B vitamins, research shows that certain types of fish may contain dangerous levels of mercury. Nearly all fish and shellfish contain traces of *methylmercury*, a type of mercury found in water that can be harmful, especially to unborn babies and young children whose nervous systems are still developing. The risk for mercury lies in both the type of seafood consumed, as well as the amount. Through a joint consumer advisory, the FDA and the Environmental Protection Agency (EPA) warn that women who may be trying to become pregnant, pregnant women, nursing mothers, and young children should avoid the types of fish and shellfish with higher levels of mercury and eat only those that have lower levels. If you regularly eat types of fish high in methylmercury, the substance can accumulate in your blood over time. Although it is removed from the body naturally, it may take more than a year for the levels to drop significantly, which is why women who are trying to become pregnant also should avoid eating certain types of fish.

While, almost all fish and shellfish contain traces of methylmercury, larger fish that have lived longer contain the highest levels, as it accumulates over time. Avoid eating shark, swordfish, king mackerel, or tilefish because they contain high levels of mercury and pose the greatest risk. You should be eating up to twelve ounces (two average meals) a week of a variety of fish and shellfish that are lower in mercury. We offer several recipes incorporating fish in Chapter 10. Five of the most commonly eaten fish that are low in mercury are shrimp, canned light tuna, salmon, pollack, and catfish. Albacore (white) tuna has more mercury than canned light tuna. When choosing your meals of fish and shellfish, you may eat up to six ounces, one average meal, of albacore tuna per week. In addition, you should check to see if advisories exist concerning the safety of fish caught in local lakes, rivers, and coastal areas. If no advice is available, eat up to six ounces per week of fish you catch from local waters, but don't consume any other fish during that week.

What Are Carbohydrates?

Carbohydrates are produced by photosynthesis in plants and are the primary source of energy found in plant foods including fruits, vegetables, grains, legumes, and tubers. Carbohydrates have an important role in the functioning of the internal organs, nervous system, and muscles and are the best source of energy for endurance athletics because they provide both an immediate and time-released energy source. These compounds are needed to regulate protein and fat metabolism, as well as help to fight infections, promote growth, and lubricate the joints.

Once grouped into two main categories, simple carbs included sugars—such as fruit sugar (fructose), corn or grape sugar (dextrose or glucose), and table sugar (sucrose)—while complex carbs included everything made of three or more linked sugars. In the digestive system, carbohydrates are broken down into single sugar molecules that are then absorbed into the bloodstream and used as energy.

Not All Carbs Are Created Equal

It's a shame that the entire carbohydrate family gets a bad rap for their delinquent stripped cousins. The naked truth of the matter is that when the integrity of whole grains is preserved, the effects on health are nothing short of wholesome.

Traditionally, it has been assumed that complex carbohydrates cause smaller rises in blood sugar than do simple carbohydrates. A growing body of evidence, however, contradicts this notion. In fact, white bread and potatoes are digested almost immediately to glucose, causing blood sugar to rapidly spike—refuting the theory that complex carbohydrates are different from simple sugars in terms of their effects on blood sugar levels. A new system that had been embraced by the scientific community, called the *glycemic index* (*GI*), rates foods according to how fast and how far they push blood sugar, giving us a better indication of how carb-rich foods affect health.

It has been shown that the GI of a food depends on the speed of digestion and absorption into the body, which is largely determined by both its physical and chemical properties. Typically, foods with less starch to gelatinize, or form a jelly, (such as pasta) and those containing a high level of soluble fiber (such as whole-grain barley, oats, and rye), have slower rates of digestion and lower GI values. Another important factor on GI values is the ratio of a compound called *amylose* to a fiber called *amylopectin*. Foods with a higher amylose to amylopectin ratio, such as legumes and parboiled rice, tend to have lower GI values, because of the compact structure of amylase, which blunts the effects of enzymatic reactions. Conversely, amylopectin is a branched compound—making it more available to enzymatic attack in the body —promoting digestion. Use of the GI has shown that many complex carbohydrates (such as the white bread and potatoes noted) cause endocrine responses that rival pure glucose, further casting doubt on the usefulness of the simple versus complex classification system.

The principal argument against the GI concept is that it cannot tell the entire story, as blood sugar levels are influenced by both the quantity and the quality (GI rating) of the carbohydrate. In response to this concern, the concept of *glycemic load* (*GL*) was introduced. Defined as the product of the GI value of a food and its carbohydrate content, GL incorporates both the quality and quantity of carbohydrate consumed.

With white bread used as the reference standard for glycemic load, dietary GL quantifies the glucose-raising potential of dietary carbohydrates, with each unit of dietary GL representing the equivalent glycemic effect of 1 gram of carbohydrate from white bread. In general, carbohydrate-dense foods with low fiber content have high GI and GL values, including potatoes, refined cereal products, and many sugar-sweetened beverages; whereas whole grains, fruits, and vegetables with high fiber content provide low to very low GLs per serving. It should be noted, however, that many low GI foods are not necessarily high in fiber (such as pasta, basmati rice, and dairy products); whereas some high-fiber, whole-meal bread and cereal products are high in GI.

Valuable research in recent years has offered additional insight into how carbohydrates affect our endocrine system, including insulin and inflammatory processes, as well as hunger, overeating, and weight gain.

Refined Versus Whole Carbohydrates. When it became common practice to refine the wheat flour for bread by milling it, and discarding the bran and germ, consumers lost a myriad of health protective nutrients. In the 1940s, Congress passed legislation requiring that all grain products that cross state lines be enriched with iron, thiamin, riboflavin, and niacin. In 1996, this legislation was amended to include folate, because of its important role in preventing birth defects. Although enrichment—the process of adding nutrients to a food to meet a specific standard—restores and raises many of the nutrients lost during refining, recent research shows that the health consequences cannot be compensated for by adding individual nutrients back to a refined grain product for several reasons.

First, by removing the germ and bran layers of a grain, a naturally low GI food is turned into a high GI one. The fibrous coating serves to slow digestion, keeping blood sugar on an even keel. Also, the surface area is increased with refined grain products, enhancing digestive enzyme processes. As we discussed previously, this is an important element to keeping insulin and IGF levels low and maintaining a healthy weight.

Second, many nutrients in the germ and bran layers are not added back to the refined grain product, or the body poorly absorbs them. This is especially true of minerals, which are not as well absorbed from enriched foods as from naturally occurring sources. Magnesium—which has an important role in insulin function—and zinc—a mineral important for a healthy immune system—are two to note.

Third, the "New Nutritional Frontier" is still in its infancy, and we have yet to identify all of the health-protective compounds in every food. When we alter a food from its natural state, by refining for example, we may be removing a cocktail of phytonutrients and other compounds that protect us from disease.

Carbohydrate Choices and Your Weight

Because of their high fiber and water content, whole-grain foods contain fewer calories gram for gram than the same amount of corresponding refined grain food. The Nurses' Health Study (NHS) showed that women with the greatest increase in intake of whole grains gained an average of 1.52 kilograms less than did those with the smallest increase in intake of whole-grain foods. In addition, women with the highest consumption of whole grains had a 49 percent lower risk of major weight gain than did women with the highest consumption of refined grains. Researchers believe that the insulin-elevating effects of high-GI foods promote weight gain by directing nutrients away from use in muscles and toward storage in fat cells.

Almost every study conducted on the effects of carbohydrates on appetite has shown that low-GI foods (as seen in Table 4.2 on page 50) produce a feeling of satiety, or satisfaction, for a longer period of time than do their high GI counterparts (as seen in Table 4.4 on page 52). One study found both lower levels of blood sugar and a slower return of hunger after meals with a bean-based dish (low GI) versus a potato dish (high GI).

Carbohydrate Choices and Diabetes

The Framingham Research Study conducted at the Jean Mayer U.S. Department of Agriculture, Human Nutrition Research Center on Aging at Tufts University, examined the relationship between whole grains and metabolic risk factors for type 2 diabetes and cardiovascular disease. Using 2,941 participants, the study found an inverse association between whole-grain intake and fasting insulin, specifically among overweight participants.

A Harvard study looked at the intake of whole versus refined grains among 75,521 women free of diabetes and heart disease. The study determined that the women who included the most whole grains into their diet substantially reduced the risk of diabetes, especially among women with a body mass index (BMI) greater than 25. (Refer back to Chapter 2 to determine your own BMI.)

A study conducted at the University of Minnesota had similar findings. This study examined the relationship between carbohydrates, fiber, magnesium, and the glycemic index with the incidence of diabetes among 35,988 Iowa women. The study concluded that whole grains, cereal fiber, and dietary magnesium have a protective role in the development of diabetes.

The Insulin Resistance Atherosclerosis Study (IRAS) evaluated specific dietary patterns and their relationship with insulin resistance and found those participants consuming the most whole grains, specifically in the form of dark breads, had increased insulin sensitivity. Researchers believe the fiber and magnesium found in whole grains may be to credit for the beneficial effects on insulin function.

Carbs in the Kitchen

Now that we've set the stage for understanding how carbohydrates affect the cancer process, let's put it into practice! Here we offer information on classifying carbs, show you how easy it is to clean up your carb act, and give you practical pairings to get your good carbs and good fats, deliciously.

Classifying Carbs

While certain fruits, such as watermelon and carrots, are high on the GI scale, they should not be avoided because of their abundance of phytonutrients, fiber, and other compounds. However,

TABLE 4.2 Low GI Foods (Less Than 55)

Product	Food
Breads and bakery	Pumpernickel Heavy mixed grain
Breakfast cereals	All-Bran cereal Toasted muesli Psyllium-based cereal Oatmeal (old-fashioned)
Dairy foods	Milk, full fat Soy milk Milk, skim Yogurt, low-fat, fruit
Fruits and vegetables	Grapefruit Peach Apple Pear Orange Grapes Kiwi Banana Sweet potato
Rice, grains, and pastas	Fettuccini Whole-wheat spaghetti Spaghetti Long-grain rice Bulgur
Legumes	Peanuts Soybeans Lentils Chickpeas Baked beans (canned)

TABLE 4.3 **Moderate GI Foods (55–69)**	
Product	**Food**
Breads and bakery	Sourdough
	Pita bread
	Barley bread
	Rye bread
	Whole-wheat bread
Breakfast cereals	Quick-cooking oatmeal
	Cream of Wheat
	Muesli
Dairy foods	Ice cream, full fat
Fruits and vegetables	Pineapple
	Popcorn
	Pawpaw
Rice, grains, and pastas	Brown rice
	Linguine
	White Rice

aim to stock your pantry with low GI foods and enjoy them often. Look at Tables 4.2, 4.3, and 4.4 to start stocking up on an appropriate balance of low, moderate, and high GI foods.

Clean Up Your Carb Act!

Small changes can make a big impact on your health. The following list offers some helpful suggestions for replacing the carbs higher on the glycemic index with some lower alternatives.

❖ Instead of white bread, try pumpernickel or dark, whole-grain breads.
❖ Instead of white rice, try basmati rice, or Lundberg rice.

TABLE 4.4 **High GI Foods (Higher Than 69)**	
Product	**Food**
Breads and bakery	French bread
	Pretzels
	Wholemeal bread
	White bread
Breakfast cereals	Cornflakes
	Toasted whole-grain cereal such as Cheerios
	Rice cereal
Fruits and vegetables	Parsnips
	Potatoes
	Watermelon
	Carrots
Rice, grains, and pastas	Low amylase rice

* Instead of sugary breakfast cereal, try muesli, steel-cut oats, or an all-bran cereal.
* Instead of pretzels, try popcorn.
* Instead of potatoes, try beans or whole-grain pasta
* Instead of white crackers, try whole-grain rye or wheat crackers.
* Instead of cakes, light muffins, or pastries, try bran muffins or use whole-grain mixes.

Perfect Pairings

Here are some ideas from Healing Gourmet on getting a daily dose of those good fats and carbs without sacrificing taste! For more ideas on perfect pairings for balanced health, see Chapters 9 and 10, and visit our website healinggourmet.com.

* Pepperidge Farm German Dark Wheat bread with all-natural peanut butter for whole grains, PUFAs, and low GI legumes
* Ryvita Dark Rye crackers and hummus for whole grains, low-GI legumes, and MUFAs
* Grilled wild salmon and Lundberg Wehani Rice for omega-3s and whole grains
* Stonyfield Farms Black Cherry Yogurt and ground flax for low-GI carbs and omega-3s

Feast on Fiber: Bulk Is Better

One of the diabetes-beating properties of whole-grain, carbohydrate-rich foods is their abundance of fiber—an important non-nutritive compound for health that helps to keep blood sugar balanced and sweeps cholesterol out of the body.

There are two general categories of fiber: soluble and insoluble. Soluble fibers, which are easily digested, can be divided into three major types: *pectins* (found in root vegetables, cabbage, apples, whole-wheat bran, and beans), *gums* (which can be obtained from oatmeal, dried beans, and other legumes), and *mucilages* (which are synthesized by plant cells and are found in food additives).

There are also several types of insoluble fibers. *Cellulose* can be found in cabbage, peas, apples, root vegetables, whole-wheat flour, beans, bran, and wheat. *Hemicellulose* is found in bran, cereals, and whole grains. *Lignan*, most abundantly found in flaxseed, is a phytonutrient that works very much like an insoluble fiber. Fiber is actually classified as a carbohydrate. and in the United States the total carbohydrates listed on a food label will include dietary fiber—although it is listed separately. Insoluble fiber is also important to regulate gastrointestinal functions and to keep the colon clean.

Research studies confirm, and it is the position of the American Dietetic Association, that fiber is an important element in stabilizing blood sugar, reducing cholesterol, achieving a healthy weight, and preventing the cardiovascular complications of diabetes. In particular, water-soluble fiber is beneficial for people with diabetes for several key reasons:

* It slows digestion and the absorption of nutrients, resulting in a slow and steady release of glucose from the other carbohydrates that accompany it.
* It soaks up excess bile acids found in the intestinal tract, which are converted into blood cholesterol by the body.
* It delays stomach emptying, causing a feeling of fullness or satiety that is useful in achieving or maintaining a healthy weight.

Fiber, Diabetes, and Weight Gain

Harvard studies, the Nurses' Health Study, and the Health Professionals Follow-Up Study found that a diet low in cereal fiber and rich in high-GI foods (which cause big spikes in blood sugar) more than doubled the risk of type 2 diabetes when compared to a diet high in cereal fiber and low in high-GI foods.

Another Harvard study found that weight gain among 74,091 nurses was inversely associated with high-fiber, whole-grain foods and positively associated with the intake of refined-grain foods.

Fiber, Heart Disease, and C-Reactive Protein

Getting lots of dietary fiber has been linked to a lower risk of heart disease in a number of large studies that followed people for many years. In a Harvard study of more than 40,000 male health professionals, researchers found that a high total dietary-fiber intake was linked to a 40 percent lower risk of coronary heart disease, compared to a low-fiber intake.

In the Nurses' Health Study, which involved nearly 69,000 women in a ten-year follow-up investigation, researchers found that fiber obtained from eating cereals, vegetables, and fruit lowered cardiovascular heart disease risk. Increased consumption of cereal grains conferred the greatest benefit.

A recent study conducted at the Centers for Disease Control and Prevention examined the association between dietary fiber and serum concentration of C-reactive protein (CRP). Using data from the National Health and Nutrition Examination Survey 1999–2000, which evaluated the diets of 3,920 participants, the study concluded that dietary-fiber intake was inversely associated with serum CRP concentration.

Getting the Most

The American Diabetes Association (ADA) recommends 20 to 35 grams of fiber daily for all adults. Clinical studies have shown that up to 50 grams of fiber per day can improve glycemic control and reduce lipid levels in people with type 2 diabetes. The ADA also says that people with type 1 or type 2 diabetes who have abnormal cholesterol levels can benefit from 10 to 25 grams of soluble fiber daily. Table 4.5 summarizes some general sources of fiber. Remember to increase the amount of both kinds of fiber. Here are some tips to help you get a good balance.

❖ Choose fresh fruit or vegetables rather than juice.
❖ Eat the skin and membranes of cleaned fruits and vegetables.
❖ Choose bran and whole-grain breads and cereals daily.
❖ When you increase fiber you should also increase your water intake.

TABLE 4.5 **Fiber Content of Selected Foods**

Food Item	Total(g)	Soluble(g)	Insoluble(g)
Legumes			
Chickpeas (½ cup)	6.2	1.3	4.9
Kidney beans (½ cup cooked)	5.8	2.9	2.9
Navy beans (½ cup cooked)	5.8	2.2	3.6
Northern beans (½ cup)	5.6	1.4	4.2
Pinto beans (½ cup cooked)	7.4	1.9	5.5
Soybeans (½ cup cooked)	5.1	2.3	2.8
Tofu (½ cup)	1.4	0.9	0.6
Cereal Grains			
Barley (½ cup, cooked)	4.2	0.9	3.3
Bulgur (½ cup, cooked)	2.9	0.5	2.4
Couscous (½ cup, cooked)	1.3	0.3	1.0
Millet (½ cup, cooked)	3.3	0.6	2.7
Noodles (spinach, ½ cup)	0.9	0.4	0.5
Noodles (white spaghetti)	0.9	0.4	0.5
Noodles (whole wheat)	2.3	0.5	1.8

Rice, brown (½ cup, cooked)	1.7	0.1	1.6
Rice, white (½ cup, cooked)	0.2	0	.2
Rice, wild (½ cup, cooked)	1.5	0.2	1.3
Breads (1 medium slice)			
Multigrain	1.8	0.3	1.5
Pita (7″-diameter, wheat)	4.4	0.7	3.7
Pumpernickel	1.5	0.8	0.7
Rye	1.5	0.8	0.7
Tortilla (6″-diameter, plain)	1.4	0.2	1.1
Tortilla (8″-diameter, plain)	1.4	0.4	1.0
White or sourdough	0.7	0.4	0.3
Whole wheat	1.9	0.3	1.6
Cereal (1 cup)			
All-Bran	10	1	9
Bran cereal with raisins	8.4	1.2	7.2
Cornflakes	0.7	0	0.7
Farina	1.2	0.5	0.7
Grits, corn	0.4	0	0.4

(continued)

TABLE 4.5 *(continued)*

Food Item	Total(g)	Soluble(g)	Insoluble(g)
Cereal (continued)			
Oatmeal	3.8	1.8	2.0
Toasted whole-grain cereal (such as Cheerios)	2.6	1.2	1.4
Snacks			
Popcorn (light, 3 cups)	2.3	0	2.3
Popcorn (microwave, 3 cups)	2.4	0	2.4
Fruits (fresh)			
Apple (3"-diameter)	5.7	1.5	4.2
Applesauce (½ cup)	1.6	0.5	1.1
Banana (7"-long)	2.8	0.7	2.1
Blackberries (½ cup)	3.8	3.1	0.7
Blueberries (½ cup)	1.9	0.2	1.7
Cherries (fresh, ½ cup)	1.7	0.5	1.2
Figs (3 small)	5.3	2.3	3.0
Grapefruit (half, 4"-diameter)	1.5	1.2	0.3

Grapes (½ cup)	0.8	0.3	0.5
Juice (apple, 6 oz)	0.2	0.1	0.1
Juice (orange, 6 oz)	0.4	0.2	0.2
Kiwi (large)	3.1	0.7	2.4
Mango (medium)	3.7	1.5	2.2
Melon (⅕ of 6″-diameter)	0.7	0.2	0.5
Orange (3″-diameter)	4.4	2.6	1.8
Peach (medium)	3.2	1.3	1.9
Pear (3″-diameter)	4.0	2.2	1.8
Pineapple (½ cup)	1.0	0.1	0.9
Plum (large)	1.7	0.9	0.8
Prunes (3 medium)	1.9	1.0	0.9
Raisins (¼ cup)	1.5	0.4	1.1
Raspberries (½ cup)	4.2	0.4	3.8
Strawberries (½ cup)	1.9	0.5	1.4
Vegetables			
Artichoke (medium, cooked)	6.5	4.7	1.8
Asparagus spears (cooked)	1.4	0.7	0.7

(continued)

TABLE 4.5 *(continued)*

Food Item	Total(g)	Soluble(g)	Insoluble(g)
Vegetables *(continued)*			
Beans (cooked, ½ cup)	1.9	0.8	1.1
Beets (½ cup)	1.5	0.7	0.8
Beets (½ cup)	1.5	0.7	0.8
Bok choy (cooked ½ cup)	1.4	0.5	0.9
Bok choy (raw, 1 cup)	0.7	0.3	0.4
Broccoli (cooked)	1.4	1.2	1.2
Broccoli (raw, ½ cup)	1.3	0.5	0.8
Brussels sprouts (½ cup)	3.3	2.0	1.3
Cabbage (green, cooked)	1.8	0.8	1.0
Cabbage (red, shredded)	0.8	0.3	0.5
Carrots (baby, 6)	2.8	1.4	1.4
Carrots (cooked, ½ cup)	1.6	1.1	1.5
Cauliflower (cooked, ½ cup)	1.7	0.4	1.3
Cauliflower (raw, ½ cup)	1.3	0.5	0.8
Celery (1 large stalk)	1.1	0.4	0.7
Chiles (hot pepper, raw)	3.0	1.5	1.5

Corn (½ cup)	2.0	0.3	1.7
Eggplant, cooked (½ cup)	1.3	0.4	0.9
Greens (cooked, ½ cup)	0.4	0.1	0.3
Jicama (raw, ½ cup)	3.2	1.7	1.5
Lettuce (Iceberg, 1 cup)	0.8	0.1	0.7
Lettuce (Romaine, 1 cup)	0.9	0.3	0.6
Frozen single or mixed vegetables (½ cup)			
Broccoli and cauliflower	1.5	0.6	0.9
Broccoli, peppers, and mushrooms	1.8	0.7	1.1
Corn, green beans, and carrots	4.0	1.9	2.1
Lima beans and corn	4.9	1.8	3.1
Mushrooms (cooked, sliced)	1.8	0.2	1.6
Onions (½ cup cooked)	2.0	1.2	0.8
Peas (cooked, ½ cup)	4.3	1.2	3.1
Peas and carrots	2.5	0.9	1.6
Peppers (green and red, ½ cup)	1.3	0.5	0.8
Potato (mashed, ½ cup)	1.6	0.9	0.7
Potato (with skin, medium)	2.9	1.2	1.7

(continued)

TABLE 4.5 *(continued)*

Food Item	Total(g)	Soluble(g)	Insoluble(g)
Frozen single mixed vegetables (½ cup) *(continued)*			
Pumpkin (mashed, ½ cup)	3.6	0.5	3.1
Spinach (cooked, ½ cup)	2.7	0.5	2.2
Spinach (raw, 1 cup)	0.4	0.1	0.3
Squash (butternut)	1.7	0.7	1.0
Squash (winter, cooked)	3.3	1.9	1.4
Sweet potatoes (½ cup)	3.8	1.4	2.4
Tomatoes (medium, raw)	0.9	0	0.9
Water chestnuts (½ cup)	1.2	0.9	1.3
Zucchini (cooked, ½ cup)	1.2	0.5	0.7

* Eat fewer processed foods and more fresh ones, as processing often removes fiber.
* Try to get fiber from foods rather than fiber supplements, as foods are more nutritious and supply an array of health-promoting phytonutrients.

Love Your Legumes

The evidence for beans to benefit diabetes and heart disease is so strong that we're devoting a section to get you to love your legumes! Beans are a low-GI food and an excellent source of fiber —making them a smart choice for people concerned with diabetes, weight control, and heart disease.

Beans release sugar slowly into the bloodstream ensuring blood sugar stays stable. The insoluble fiber causes the body to produce more insulin receptor sites—tiny "docks" that insulin molecules latch onto—meaning more insulin gets into cells where it is needed and less is present in the bloodstream where it can cause problems. The low GI of beans has been attributed to many factors including their fiber, tannin, and phytic acid contents.

Beans also help to keep cholesterol low, a main component in the risk of cardiovascular disease, which is prevalent in diabetes. Compounds, including *saponins* and *phytoestrogens*, may be to credit for the cholesterol-lowering benefits of beans. Saponins, a naturally occurring compound found in legumes, combine with lipids and form soaplike foams that carry cholesterol out of the body. Saponins decrease blood lipids, lower cancer risks, and reduce blood sugar.

Phytoestrogens, including isoflavones found primarily in soybeans, have been found to improve glucose control and insulin resistance, as well as reduce cholesterol. Researchers believe these compounds modulate the secretion of insulin from the pancreas and also act as antioxidants.

Kitchen Prescription

Balance your blood sugar with beans in our delicious recipes including Lemon Garbanzo Soup, Bean and Veggie Soup, Crunchy Lentil Salad, Spicy Noodles Salad with Baked Tofu, or Asian Tofu Cakes.

Now that you have some ideas for balancing the good and bad fats and carbohydrates, plus getting a healthy dose of fiber and learning to love your legumes, it's time to look at the benefits of increasing your intake of antioxidants and phytonurients, as well as how to incorporate these important foods into your diet.

Antioxidants, Phytonutrients, and Other Diabetes-Fighting Nutrients

INDIVIDUAL COMPOUNDS in foods are getting special attention for their honorable actions as defenders of our health. These antioxidants and phytonutrients join forces like players on a football team to balance our blood sugar, reduce inflammation, and keep cholesterol levels in check. Just as the quarterback alone can't win the game, no single nutrient has the ability to conquer disease. In this chapter, we'll discuss the lineup of team players and their position on the field of health for a diabetes-beating nutritional strategy.

Free Radical Defense

In the fight against diabetes, the free radical rival makes about 10,000 attacks every day. These unstable oxygen molecules have lost an electron and, like a sneaky opponent, move swiftly through the playing field of your body, trying to steal electrons from other molecules. This in turn creates more free radicals and leaves damaged cells in the wake. Some free radicals arise normally during metabolism, but environmental factors such as pollution, poor food choices, radiation, cigarette smoke, and herbicides can also generate free radicals.

Our defensive line, including our immune system and antioxidants produced by the liver (such as glutathione and superoxide dismutase), needs fuel from outside sources to conquer our health-robbing adversary. Quite simply, the fuel is food, and good dietary decisions tip the odds in a victory against diabetes.

Diabetes: An Increased Need to Fight Free Radicals

Hyperglycemia, or high blood sugar, has been found to be responsible for much of the oxidative stress in diabetes, which is a key factor in diabetic complications including heart disease and problems with the nerves and eyes. Research shows that balancing blood sugar and incorporating antioxidants into the diet may help to reduce oxidant stress and complications of diabetes. Free radicals have been found to have detrimental effects on the function of many cells including:

❖ Insulin-secreting beta cells of the pancreas
❖ Fat cells
❖ Muscle cells
❖ Nerve cells

As high blood sugar worsens, the insulin-producing beta cells of the pancreas steadily deteriorate, secrete less and less insulin, and lose function. In type 1 diabetes, the body produces more of those inflammatory compounds called cytokines we discussed in Chapter 3 in response to the free radical foes. In type 2 diabetes, high blood sugar increases levels of damaging peroxide in the cells that secrete insulin, causing a slow death. Because of this, antioxidants have been proposed as protectors from diabetic complications.

A study published in the journal *Diabetes Care* evaluated the diets of more than 4,000 men and women between the ages of 40 and 69 who were free of diabetes at the start of the study. Researchers tracked the amounts of vitamin E, vitamin C, carotenoids, as well as other forms of vitamin E, such as tocopherols. After 23 years of follow-up, the study concluded that the people eating the most carotenoid and vitamin E rich foods had a lower risk of type 2 diabetes compared with those consuming lower levels of the antioxidants.

Like players on a team, each antioxidant plays a special role in protecting cells and organs from oxidative damage. Therefore, it's important to include all the players in your diet to win the fight against diabetes. Let's take a look at some of the superstars you should have on your starting lineup.

The Antioxidant Superstars

With the evolution of technology, researchers are able to measure the levels of antioxidants in specific foods, helping us to identify the star players. Remember, digestion, absorption, and methods of cooking play a role in the amount of antioxidants in foods, so be sure to change it up and keep your diet varied. Table 5.1 summarizes the top twenty food sources of antioxidants. You'll learn

Healing Tip

Many factors affect the levels of antioxidants in foods, including the method of cooking. Some antioxidants, such as vitamin C, are water soluble; others, such as lycopene and other carotenoids, are lipid or fat soluble. In general, lipid-soluble antioxidants are best absorbed by the body when cooked and consumed with a bit of fat (oil); whereas water-soluble foods are best fresh, as cooking destroys these compounds or they are lost in the water.

TABLE 5.1 Top Twenty Food Sources of Antioxidants

Rank	Food	Serving Size	Total Antioxidant Capacity per Serving
1	Small red beans (dried)	½ cup	13,727
2	Wild blueberries	1 cup	13,427
3	Red kidney beans (dried)	½ cup	13,259
4	Pinto beans	½ cup	11,864
5	Blueberries (cultivated)	1 cup	9,019
6	Cranberries (whole)	1 cup	8,983
7	Artichoke hearts (cooked)	1 cup	7,904
8	Blackberries	1 cup	7,701
9	Dried prunes	½ cup	7,291
10	Raspberries	1 cup	6,058
11	Strawberries	1 cup	5,938
12	Red delicious apples	One	5,900
13	Granny smith apples	One	5,381
14	Pecans	1 oz.	5,095
15	Sweet cherries	1 cup	4,873
16	Black plums	One	4,844
17	Russet potatoes (cooked)	One	4,649
18	Black beans (dried)	½ cup	4,181
19	Plums	One	4,118
20	Gala apples	One	3,903

about the phytonutrients responsible for these free radical fighting actions in the next section.

Phytonutrient Fuel: A Clean Pass

Much of the good press antioxidants get is due to tiny compounds called phytonutrients found inside the fruits, vegetables, legumes, and grains. These phytonutrients ("phyto" meaning plant) protect plants against harsh weather conditions and hungry insects and even heal the wounds made by the nibbling moth. With their own defensive lineup, plant foods stand ready to guard against hungry predators trying to take a bite or fungi that hang around, draining their resources.

This plant protection system—essentially antioxidants and phytonutrients—not only serves as defense, but is also credited for the vibrant colors and delicious flavors of our food. Interestingly, distinguishing colors is a trait common only to humans and a few species of primates. So the foods most appealing to our eye are also most appealing to our body to prevent and treat diseases.

It should come as no surprise that fruits and vegetables with higher levels of antioxidants produce fresher food for longer periods of time (shelf life) with less risk of mold. These foods are better equipped to preserve and protect themselves; when we take a bite, we become the proverbial receiver of those antioxidants and phytonutrients—making a clean pass of diabetes-beating nutrients onto us.

Unfortunately, the development of agriculture some ten thousand years ago caused a shift away from our diverse plant-based diet that provides a spectrum of essential vitamins and minerals, and tens of thousands of protective phytonutrients. Replacing this delicious and defensive diet with processed foods, refined grains, and added oils, sugar, and salt has led to the rise of chronic diseases including diabetes. In fact, today most Americans eat between two and three servings of fruits and vegetables per day (when the optimum is seven to nine servings), and a minority eat none at all.

Advances in technology have allowed us to further explore compounds in foods on a molecular level, distinguishing between the thousands of plant nutrients in individual foods and food families. This "New Nutritional Frontier" provides us with critical information on how best we can use foods to balance blood sugar and prevent complications associated with diabetes. It is estimated that twenty-five thousand individual phytonutrients have been identified in fruits, vegetables, and grains; a large percentage still remain unknown and need to be identified before we can fully understand their health benefits.

Your body's multiplayer defense system is assisted by the phytonutrient fuel you feed it. Each time you eat fruits, vegetables, or other antioxidant-rich foods, you catch the pass, and a flood of diabetes-beating, heart-protecting nutrients enters your bloodstream.

The Vitamin and Mineral Team of Players

These "old school" standbys have taught us few new things in recent decades. Although we have known about the actions of vitamins and minerals for some time, only recently have we begun to understand their individual roles in diabetes. See Table 5.2 for information on serving sizes so you have a frame of reference when reviewing the following Kitchen Prescriptions.

Biotin

It has been known for many years that a biotin deficiency causes an improper use of glucose in the body. In laboratory studies, biotin has been found to stimulate the secretion of insulin, helping to reduce blood sugar.

TABLE 5.2 **Serving Size Guide**

Food Group	Serving Size	Visual Comparison
Grains	1 slice bread; ½ cup cooked cereal, rice, or pasta; 1 cup ready-to-eat cereal	½ cup cooked pasta = a scoop of ice cream; 1 cup dry cereal = a large handful
Vegetables	½ cup chopped raw or cooked veggies; 1 cup leafy raw veggies	1 cup veggies = the size of your fist
Fruits	1 medium apple, orange, or banana; ½ cup juice or canned fruit; ¼ cup dried fruit	1 medium piece of fruit = a baseball
Dairy	1 cup milk or yogurt; 2 ounces cheese	2 ounces cheese = a pair of dominos
Protein foods	3 ounces cooked lean meat, poultry, or fish; ½ cup dried beans, 1 egg counts as 1 ounce of lean meat; 2 tablespoons peanut butter	3 ounces meat or fish = the palm of your hand
Fats	1 teaspoon butter; 1 teaspoon oil	1 teaspoon butter = the tip of your thumb

Kitchen Prescription

Those low-glycemic-index, carb-rich foods we talked about in Chapter 4 supply sugar-balancing biotin. You can get it in soybeans, rice bran, peanut butter, barley, and oatmeal.

Calcium

Like magnesium, calcium helps cells to communicate with one another and plays a role in mediating the constriction and relaxation of blood vessels, nerve impulse transmission, muscle contraction, and the secretion of hormones including insulin. This common mineral has beneficial effects on lipids and may aid in weight control as well. By forming insoluble soaps with fatty acids in the intestine, calcium helps to prevent the absorption of part of the dietary fat, thus reducing cholesterol.

 Kitchen Prescription

Cut the Cholesterol! Get calcium in yogurt (415 mg or 42 percent DV), skim milk (402 mg or 30 percent DV), tofu (204 mg or 20 percent DV), orange juice (200 mg or 20 percent DV), salmon (181 mg or 18 percent DV), cooked spinach (120 mg or 12 percent DV), kale (94 mg or 9 percent DV), and bok choy (74 mg or 7 percent DV).

Magnesium

As one of the most abundant ions present in living cells, studies have shown that magnesium helps insulin get inside cells and improve their function. When there is a low concentration of magnesium inside cells, insulin receptors don't function as well, worsening insulin resistance. It is also important for heart health.

Kitchen Prescription

Magnificent Magnesium! Get it in a typical serving of halibut (90 mg or 20 percent DV), almonds (80 mg or 20 percent DV), cashews (75 mg or 20 percent DV), soybeans (75 mg or 20 percent DV), spinach (75 mg or 20 percent DV), oatmeal (55 mg or 15 percent DV), potatoes (50 mg or 15 percent DV), peanuts (50 mg or 15 percent DV), black-eyed peas (45 mg or 10 percent DV), yogurt (45 mg or 10 percent DV), baked beans (40 mg or 10 percent DV), and brown rice (40 mg or 10 percent DV).

Vitamin B₁ (Thiamin)

Vitamin B_1, or thiamin, is necessary for processing carbohydrates, fats, and protein and is also necessary for the production of adenine triphosphate (ATP), the basic unit of energy in the body. Having an important role in nerve functioning, thiamin is also an important coenzyme that assists in the metabolism of glucose.

Kitchen Prescription

Get thiamin in lentils (0.17 mg or 15 percent DV), peas (0.19 mg or 17 percent DV), brown rice (0.10 mg or 9 percent), Brazil nuts (0.17 mg or 15 percent DV), pecans (0.13 mg or 12 percent DV), spinach (0.02 mg or 2 percent DV), orange (0.05 mg or 5 percent DV), and cantaloupe (0.07 or 6 percent DV).

Vitamin B₃ (Niacin)

Vitamin B₃, or niacin, is part of *glucose tolerance factor* (*GTF*), which is important in keeping your body sensitive to insulin. A deficiency of niacin makes it difficult for your body to produce GTF, which could lead to or worsen insulin resistance. Niacin has also been found to protect against kidney disease that occurs in diabetes complications.

Kitchen Prescription

Be Sensitive to Insulin! Get niacin in chicken (9.52 mg or 68 percent DV), turkey (5.41 mg or 39 percent DV), salmon (6.68 mg or 48 percent DV), mackerel (5.83 mg or 42 percent DV), tuna (8.96 mg or 64 percent DV), barley (1.62 mg or 12 percent DV), bulgur (0.91 mg or 6 percent DV), pasta (1.56 mg or 11 percent DV), lentils (1.05 mg or 8 percent DV), dried peaches (3.5 mg or 3 percent DV), and avocados (0.63 or 4 percent DV).

Vitamins B₆ and B₁₂

Vitamins B₆ and B₁₂ help reduce levels of heart-harming homocysteine (Hcy), which, as previously discussed in Chapter 3, is a sulfur-containing amino acid. The results of more than eighty studies indicate that even moderately elevated levels of Hcy in the blood increase the risk of cardiovascular diseases.

Kitchen Prescription

Boost your Bs! Get heart-helping vitamin B$_6$ in potatoes (0.7 mg or 35 percent DV), garbanzo beans (0.57 mg or 30 percent DV), chicken breast (0.52 mg or 25 percent DV), oatmeal (0.42 mg or 20 percent DV), trout (0.29 mg or 15 percent DV), sunflower seeds (0.23 mg or 10 percent DV), avocadoes (0.20 mg or 10 percent DV), tuna (0.20 mg or 10 percent DV), and cooked spinach (0.14 mg or 8 percent DV). You'll find vitamin B$_{12}$ in clams (84.1 mg or 1,400 percent DV), trout (5.4 mg or 90 percent DV), salmon (4.9 mg or 80 percent DV), yogurt (1.4 mg or 25 percent DV), tuna (1 mg or 15 percent DV), and milk (0.9 mg or 15 percent DV).

Folate

Folate gets its name from the latin word *folium*, for leaf, and hence is present in good amounts in leafy greens. Folate works in conjunction with vitamin B$_6$ and vitamin B$_{12}$ to help recycle homocysteine into methionine. A number of studies have shown that high levels of homocysteine are associated with an increased risk of heart disease.

 Healing Tip

Beans and Greens! If you frequently dine on "beans and greens" you're fine with folate. You can get it in black-eyed peas (105 mcg or 25 percent DV), cooked spinach (100 mcg or 25 percent DV), great northern beans (90 mcg or 20 percent DV), asparagus (85 mcg or 20 percent DV), wheat germ (40 mcg or 10 percent DV), orange juice (35 mcg or 10 percent DV), peas (50 mcg or 15 percent DV), cooked broccoli (45 mcg or 15 percent DV), avocadoes (45 mcg or 10 percent DV), and peanuts (40 mcg or 10 percent DV).

Vitamin C (Ascorbic Acid)

Vitamin C, or ascorbic acid, is a water-soluble vitamin. As we discussed earlier in the chapter, antioxidant nutrients have important roles in reducing free radical damage associated with diabetes and cardiovascular disease, as well as macular degeneration, cataracts, asthma, and many other chronic illnesses.

 Kitchen Prescription

Orange You Healthy? Get your daily dose of vitamin C in oranges (78 mg or 104 percent DV), grapefruit (132 mg or 178 percent DV), blueberries (14 mg or 19 percent DV), strawberries (122 mg or 163 percent DV), mangoes (57 mg or 76 percent DV), papaya (94 mg or 125 percent DV), cantaloupe (70 mg or 93 percent DV), watermelon (12 mg or 16 percent DV), sweet potato (18 mg or 24 percent DV), green peppers (95 mg or 125 percent DV), and red peppers (226 mg or 301 percent DV).

Vitamin E (Alpha Tocopherol)

As a fat-soluble antioxidant vitamin, vitamin E, or alpha tocopherol, may protect against the free radical damage associated with diabetes, as well as help reduce the cardiovascular complications. Some evidence suggests vitamin E may also promote healing of diabetic wounds and promote healing.

Kitchen Prescription

Es to Please! Vitamin E is found in wheat germ oil (20.3 mg or 100 percent DV), almonds (7.4 mg or 40 percent DV), sunflower seeds (6 mg or 40 percent DV), hazelnuts (4.3 mg or 20 percent DV), peanuts (2.2 mg or 10 percent DV), mangoes (0.9 mg or 6 percent DV), broccoli (1.2 mg or 6 percent DV), spinach (1.6 mg or 6 percent DV), and kiwi (1.1 mg or 6 percent DV).

The Phytonutrient Team of Players

Don't let the big names of these tiny compounds scare you. They deliver a powerful diabetes-beating punch even when you don't call them by name. The important thing to do to eat to beat diabetes is to include the full spectrum—everyday!

Phenolic Phytonutrients and Flavonoids

Phenolics represent a very large category of more than two thousand phytonutrients. The term *phenol* comes from the chemical structure of these phytonutrients that vary from having one to several powerful phenol groups, which have the ability to sweep up many free radicals as they circulate through the bloodstream. This reduces damage to cells and oxidation of LDL cholesterol. Considered to be some of the most powerful antioxidants, phenolics are being studied for their ability to slow the aging process and also have anti-inflammatory, heart-protective, and clot-busting, effects. Let's take a look at the phenolic family and how each member allies forces for your health.

Flavonoids are molecular compounds found only in plants, which serve as a defense mechanism. Because plants don't have the fight-or-flight option that animals do, they must protect themselves chemically; flavonoids make the plant tissue unappetizing to fungi, insects, and other organisms harmful to plants. Every plant makes flavonoids, but they tend to be concentrated in the leaves and fruit. Therefore, fruits tend to be a richer source of flavonoids than many vegetables. Dietary flavonoids have been found to repair a range of oxidative radical damages on DNA, which can contribute to disease and the ravages of aging.

 Kitchen Prescription

Fabulous flavonoids can be found in apples, broccoli, celery, citrus fruits, cocoa, eggplants, endive, grapes, grapefruit, leeks, onion, parsley, raspberries, red wine, strawberries, and tea.

Tannins. These substances, primarily found in tea, have been studied for their actions on inflammation and their ability to kill viruses and bacteria. Intake of five flavonoids—the majority of which was derived from tannins in tea—was found to be inversely associated with dying from cardiovascular disease, a major complication of diabetes.

 Kitchen Prescription

Drink to Your Health! Get tannins in green tea, oolong tea, black tea, sorghum, red wine, and coffee.

Anthocyanins. These brightly colored compounds have recently been found to have beneficial effects on fat by reducing their secretion of inflammatory cytokines.

Kitchen Prescription

Berry Delicious Medicine! You can find these compounds most readily in red-blue fruits, including blueberries, raspberries, lingonberries, cherries, currants, pomegranate, strawberries, concord grapes, cranberries, and elderberries. Buy them frozen, and add to smoothies or thaw for a quick addition to cereal.

Quercetin. This naturally occurring antioxidant helps to beat diabetes and protect the heart. A recent study conducted at the National Public Health Institute in Helsinki, Finland, studied the association between flavonoids and several chronic diseases. The study examined the dietary intakes of 10,054 men and women consuming flavonoids in Finnish foods. The study found a trend in reduction of type 2 diabetes with the intake of quercetin and myricetin, possibly because of their beneficial effects on the kidneys and antioxidant action.

 Kitchen Prescription

Don't Quit the Quercetin! You can get quercetin in red grapes, red and yellow onions, broccoli, and apples.

Isoflavones. Isoflovones are *phytoestrogens* (plant estrogens) that help to reduce cholesterol and benefit diabetes. Numerous isoflavones exist including daidzein, genistein, and glycitein. The FDA says that 25 grams of soy protein as part of a diet low in saturated fat and cholesterol may reduce the risk of heart disease. As we discussed earlier, glucose causes LDL to be oxidized, which contributes to heart disease. Studies show that soy, because of isoflavones such as genistein, is useful in preventing heart disease, improving cholesterol levels, and producing an antidiabetic effect.

 Kitchen Prescription

Oh Soy! Get a daily dose of isoflavones in soy products such as tofu, soy milk, and edamame.

Lignans. As a phytoestrogen, lignans have been found to be beneficial in facilitating weight loss and benefiting diabetes. Researchers believe that lignans act as antioxidants and also enhance the function of insulin.

 Kitchen Prescription

Get the Flax! Lignans are found in high concentrations in flaxseed and in olive oil as well as in legumes including peas, beans, and lentils. To get the maximum benefit of lignans buy whole flaxseed and grind them in a coffee grinder. Sprinkle over cereal or yogurt, add to smoothies, or bake into whole-grain baked goods.

Curcumin. Credited for the unique flavors and golden color of curries, curcumin has potent antioxidant activity. This spicy phytonutrient may help to reduce blood sugar and protect the kidneys by reducing blood cholesterol levels.

Kitchen Prescription

Spicy Protection! Curcumin is found in turmeric, and you can get the benefits of this amazing phytonutrient with our recipe for Indian Spice Mix.

Indian Spice Mix
2 teaspoons ground turmeric
8 teaspoons dry mustard
4 teaspoons ground fenugreek
4 teaspoons ground cumin
2 teaspoons ground ginger
2 teaspoons ground coriander
2 teaspoons ground cloves
½ teaspoons ground cinnamon

Combine all ingredients in a small bowl with an airtight lid. Shake well to blend. Store in a cool dry place, sealed. Add to chicken, fish, and bean dishes.

Makes about 24½ teaspoons

Gingerols. These aromatic phytonutrients are found in—what else?—ginger! This compound, along with others in the ginger family, have been found to improve insulin sensitivity and prevent the oxidation of LDL cholesterol.

 Kitchen Prescription

Add Some Zing! Ginger is a member of the *Zingiberaceae* family, which also includes turmeric. Try our Gingered Green Tea Cooler found in Chapter 10.

Carotenoid Phytonutrients

Carotenoids, a group of more than six hundred related nutrients, have received substantial attention both because of their provitamin and antioxidant roles. Results from the Third National Health and Nutrition Examination Survey, conducted by the Centers for Disease Control and Prevention, found that carotenoids in the diet are inversely associated with fasting serum insulin. Carotenoids are also known to protect the heart. Researchers agree that getting the spectrum of carotenoids is the best strategy to improve your health and get their maximum antioxidant benefits.

 Kitchen Prescription

Fourteen-Carrot Protection! As fat-soluble compounds, you can get the most protection by cooking these foods and adding a little oil. It helps make the phytonutrients more available to your body so more gets into your bloodstream to fend off diabetes.

Lycopene. Lycopene is well known for its ability to protect the heart by reducing the oxidation of LDL cholesterol.

 Kitchen Prescription

Love Your Lycopene! Other than tomatoes, you can get lycopene in watermelons, guavas, papaya, apricots, pink grapefruit, and blood oranges. It's fat soluble too, so cook those tomatoes well, add some extra-virgin olive oil, and toss with your favorite pasta!

Lutein and Zeaxanthin. These antioxidant carotenoids are most famous for their role in reducing the risk of age-related macular degeneration. A Harvard study found that these two phytonutrients also help to decrease the risk of cataracts.

 Kitchen Prescription

Outta Sight! Get lutein and zeaxanthin in broccoli, kale, spinach, and egg yolks.

Organosulfur Compounds

Mainly found in the broccoli (*Cruciferae*) family of vegetables, organosulfur compounds have potent antioxidant activity and are best known for their ability to fight cancer. Because of the oxidative stress that occurs with diabetes, coupled with the cancer-promoting properties of insulin, people with diabetes are at an increased risk for hormone-dependent cancers. In this family of phytonutrients you will find isothiocyanates, indoles, and several others.

 Kitchen Prescription

Cellular Defense! Eat your cruciferous veggies for their potent antioxidant action. Get these fabulous phytonutrients in vegetables including broccoli, cauliflower, cabbage, kale, watercress, collards, and radishes.

Allylic Sulfur Compounds

Derived mainly from the allium, or onion, family, these phytonutrients give the characteristic bite to onions, garlic, and other relatives of this bulb group. These compounds have been found to protect the heart, stabilize blood sugar, and fight cancer.

Ajoene is a compound found in garlic and is known for its blood-thinning and cholesterol-lowering properties.

Allicin is a compound formed in garlic when an intact clove of garlic is crushed. An odorless amino acid, alliin is enzymatically converted by allinase into allicin when the cloves are crushed. Allicin is thought to be one of the most biologically active compounds in garlic protecting LDL cholesterol against oxidation and preventing the complications associated with diabetes.

Sulfides are also found in garlic as well as in cabbage, broccoli, brussels sprouts, and other members of the crucifer family. Diallyl disulfide (DADS), a substance that is formed from the compounds present in garlic, is known to increase levels of detoxifying enzymes in the body, including glutathione. Sulfides act as antithrombotic compounds (clot busters) and may protect against heart disease and strokes by thinning the blood, preventing oxidation of LDL cholesterol and reducing blood pressure.

Kitchen Prescription

Cloves of Protection! Don't let anyone tell you garlic breath isn't beautiful. Crush it and mix in with a simple dressing of extra-virgin olive oil and balsamic vinegar and drizzle over a big mixed green salad full of phytonutrients or enjoy it in our recipe for Garlicky Bruschetta.

Garlicky Bruschetta
4 tomatoes, chopped
4 garlic cloves, crushed
½ shallot, diced
½ cup fresh basil, chopped
¼ cup extra-virgin olive oil
8 slices whole-grain Italian bread, sliced

Mix all diabetes-crushing ingredients together (except bread). Let stand for 10 minutes. Toast whole-grain bread and top with tomato mixture for a dose of ajoene, allicin, sulfides, and lycopene.

Serves 8 (serving size: 1 slice bread with ¼ cup tomato mixture)

Now that you have learned about the spectrum of diabetes-beating nutrients, fats, and carbohydrates, the next chapter examines the individual foods that work together—in synergy—to help prevent and manage diabetes and stave off heart disease and other complications.

Diabetes-Beating Foods

EACH FRUIT, VEGETABLE, legume, or grain—like a team player or a note in a symphony—adds a nutritional element valuable to managing your diabetes and preventing complications. Some people are under the dangerous misconception that the cost of bad diet can be offset by taking nutritional supplements. *Wrong!* Many phytonutrients have yet to be identified. In addition, other elements, such as fiber, good fats, and the like, aren't in those pills, so you end up fighting the battle against diabetes with the wrong weapons.

The Synergy of Foods

With the diligent work of scientists worldwide and the evolution of technology, we have isolated and identified approximately twenty-five thousand unique phytonutrients in hundreds of different types of plant foods. Through research, we're learning that by combining these foods, the bioactive compounds work together—or synergistically—to increase health benefits. For example, when oranges, apples, grapes, and blueberries were tested both alone and together, the antioxidant activity was five times lower for the individual fruit than the combined fruit "salad."

Although particular groups of fruits and vegetables have been found to be especially protective for balancing blood sugar, such as legumes, research has pointed to the conclusion that diabetes management is best achieved by food synergy.

Now that you know that compounds in foods work in synergy, let's explore the families of foods and their unique blood-sugar stabilizing and heart-protective properties as seen in Table 6.1. Refer back to Chapter 5 for information on how these specific phytonutrients rally to beat diabetes.

TABLE 6.1 **Foods and Their Diabetes-Beating Properties**

Group/ Family	Foods	Phytonutrients
Cruciferae (crucifer family)	Broccoli, brussels sprouts, cabbage, cauliflower, collard greens, kale, kohlrabi, mustard greens, radishes, rutabaga, turnips, watercress	Isothiocyanates, indoles, nitriles, sulforaphane, chlorophyll
Cucurbitaceae (the melon and squash family)	Cucumbers, summer squash (pumpkin, zucchini), winter squash (acorn, butternut), cantaloupes, honeydew melons	Carotenoids, beta-carotene, alpha carotene, beta-cryptoxanthin, zeaxanthin, lutein
Labiatae (mint family)	Basil, mint, oregano, sage, rosemary, thyme	Terpenoids, menthol, chlorophyll

Leguminoseae (bean family)	Alfalfa sprouts, beans, peas, soybeans	Phytoestrogens, lignans, protease inhibitors, isoflavones, saponins
Liliaceae (lily family)	Asparagus, chives, garlic, leeks, onions, shallots	Sulfur compounds, sulfides, allicin, diallyl sulfide
Rutacea (citrus family)	Grapefruit, lemons, limes, oranges, tangerines	Limonene, carotenoids, lycopene (blood oranges and pink grapefruits), vitamin C
Solanaceae (solanum/ nightshade family)	Eggplant, peppers, potatoes, tomatoes	Lycopene, carotenoids, terpenes
Umbelliferae (umbel family)	Anise, caraway, carrots, celeriac, celery, chervil, cilantro, coriander, cumin, dill, fennel, parsley, parsnips	Carotenoids, beta-carotene, alpha carotene, beta-cryptoxanthin, zeaxanthin, lutein, chlorophyll
Zingiberaceae (ginger family)	Ginger, turmeric	Curcumin, gingerols, zingibain
Tea Family	Green tea, black tea, oolong tea, white tea varieties	Catechins, polyphenols, epigallocatechin gallate (EGCG), theaflavins

Color-Coded Cuisine

Use your plate like a canvas and paint to your heart's content! David Heber, Ph.D., of the UCLA Center for Human Nutrition in Los Angeles introduced a concept that groups foods by color to simplify eating for optimum health and disease prevention. It is not necessary to know the names of the thousands of phytonutrients present in foods to reap their health benefits. In fact, choosing a variety of foods from all of the families we have described offers the complete spectrum of nutrients needed to protect you from disease. The same phytonutrients that keep your cells healthy also give fruits and vegetables their colors and indicate their unique physiological roles. By color coding your cuisine, you can translate the science of phytonutrient nutrition into delicious dishes. The following list more closely examines what the colors mean.

❖ **Blue and purple.** Blue and purple fruits and vegetables contain varying amounts of health-promoting phytonutrients, such as anthocyanins and phenolics. Anthocyanins are currently being studied for their beneficial effects on fat cells and their ability to reduce inflammatory cytokines (previously discussed in Chapter 3).

❖ **Green.** Green vegetables contain varying amounts of phytonutrients, such as lutein and indoles, which interest researchers because of their potential antioxidant, health-promoting benefits. Lutein has an especially important role in preventing damage to the eyes, a common complication of diabetes.

❖ **White.** White, tan, and brown fruits and vegetables contain varying amounts of phytonutrients of interest to scientists. These include sulfides and allicin, found in the garlic and onion family, which help protect the heart by reducing the oxidation of LDL cholesterol.

❖ **Yellow and orange.** Yellow and orange fruits and vegetables contain varying amounts of antioxidants such as vitamin C as well as carotenoids and flavonoids. Flavonoids have a big role in protecting the heart while carotenoids play a role in reducing insulin resistance.

❖ **Red.** Lycopene and anthocyanins are the specific phytonutrients in the red group that are being studied for their health-promoting properties. Lycopene, a powerful antioxidant found in the highest concentrations in cooked tomato products, is particularly protective of the heart.

A to Z Foods: Your Diabetes-Beating Team

Balance your blood sugar deliciously! In this section, we take the colors one step further and discover the individual foods in the diabetes-beating team. We'll also show you what to look for when selecting, how to store for optimum flavor and nutritional benefits, and some recipes from Chapter 10 that incorporate these foods. Please note, that the list in this book is limited; visit our website, healinggourmet.com, for more information.

Apples

Grown in temperate zones throughout the world and cultivated for at least three thousand years, apple varieties now number well into the thousands. The apple has been called the "king of fruits," and for good reason. The quercetin found in the peel of your apples was found to reduce the occurrence of diabetes because of its antioxidant action and beneficial effects on the kidneys. These kingly fruits also provide sugar-balancing soluble fiber called *pectin* that also helps to reduce cholesterol.

✤ **Serving.** One apple (5 oz.), with skin contains 81 calories, 0.3 gram of protein, 22 grams of carbohydrate, no fat, no cholesterol, and 5 grams of dietary fiber. The same serving provides 13 percent of the RDA for vitamin C (4.8 mg), and 8 percent of the RDA for vitamin E (0.8 mg). Apples also contain phenols, chlorogenic acid, pectin, quercetin, flavonoids, boron, and salicylates.

✤ **Selecting and storing.** Available year-round, the apple's peak season is from September through November when newly harvested. Buy firm, well-colored apples with a fresh (never musty) fragrance. The skins should be smooth and free of bruises and gouges. Store apples in a cool, dark place. They do well placed in a plastic bag and stored in the refrigerator.

 Kitchen Prescription

Try our Apple and Date Muffins for a breakfast or snack that's packed with phytonutrients and diabetes-beating fiber.

Apricots

Born in China some four thousand years ago, apricots are widely consumed by the long-living Hunza people. The cousin of the peach arrived in California with the Spanish in the eighteenth century. The yellow color of these little beauties is due to carotenoids that have been found to have an inverse relation to fasting serum insulin in the Third National Health and Nutrition Examination Survey conducted by the Centers for Disease Control and Prevention.

✤ **Serving.** Three apricots (4 oz.) contain 51 calories, 1.5 grams of protein, 11.8 grams of carbohydrate, 0.5 grams of fat, no cholesterol, and 2 grams of dietary fiber. The same serving provides

28 percent of the RDA for vitamin A (200 RE), 14 percent of the RDA for vitamin C (10.5 mg), 2 percent of the RDA for iron (0.4 mg), and 272 milligrams of potassium. The apricot also contains salicylates, boron, and carotenoids.

❖ **Selecting and storing.** Because they're highly perishable and seasonal, 90 percent of the fresh apricots are marketed in June and July. When buying apricots, select plump, reasonably firm fruit with a uniform color. Store in a plastic bag in the refrigerator for three to five days.

 Kitchen Prescription

Try our Apricot and Almond Baklava, a perfect mix of carotenoids and those sugar-balancing monounsaturated fats we discussed in Chapter 4.

Artichokes

Vegetable flowers that are picked and eaten before they turn into a "real" flower, artichokes are a European staple with more than one variety. The luteolin in artichokes helps reduce cholesterol.

❖ **Serving.** One artichoke, boiled (4.2 oz.), contains 60 calories, 4.2 grams of protein, 13.4 grams of carbohydrate, 0.2 gram of fat, no cholesterol, and 6.5 grams of dietary fiber. The same serving provides 15 percent of the RDA for folate (61.2 mcg), 16 percent of the RDA for vitamin C (12 mg), 12 percent of the RDA for magnesium (47 mg), 11 percent of the RDA for iron (1.6 mg), and 425 milligrams of potassium. Artichokes also contain cynaroside, luteolin, dicaffeoylquinic, and dicaffeoyltartaric acids.

❖ **Selecting and storing.** Globe artichokes are available year-round, with the peak season from March through May. Buy deep green, heavy-for-their-size artichokes with a tight leaf formation. The leaves should "squeak" when pressed together. Heavy browning on an artichoke usually indicates it's beyond its prime. Store unwashed artichokes in a plastic bag in the refrigerator for up to four days; wash just before cooking. Artichoke hearts are available frozen and canned; artichoke bottoms are available canned.

 Kitchen Prescription

Try our Vegetarian Paella for a delicious dose of these glorious globes.

Asparagus

A member of the lily family, the edible part of asparagus is actually the young underground sprout or shoot. Asparagus provides glutathione, an antioxidant compound that may help to keep blood sugar stable and regulate blood pressure.

❖ **Serving.** One half cup of raw asparagus contains 15 calories, 1.5 grams of protein, 2.5 grams of carbohydrate, 0.1 gram of fat, no cholesterol, and 1.3 grams of dietary fiber. The same serving provides 6 percent of the RDA for vitamin A (60 RE), 48 percent of the RDA for folate (95 mcg), 37 percent of the RDA for vitamin C (22.1 mg), 5 percent of the RDA for vitamin B_6 (0.1 mg), 3 percent of the RDA for iron (0.4 mg), and 218 milligrams of potassium.

❖ **Selecting and storing.** The optimum season for fresh asparagus lasts from February through June, although hothouse asparagus is available year-round in some regions. It's best cooked the same day it's purchased but will keep, tightly wrapped in a plastic bag, for three to four days in the refrigerator. Or, store standing upright in about an inch of water, covering the container with a plastic bag.

 Kitchen Prescription

Get these spears of protection in our Pasta with Asparagus and Lemon.

Avocados

Native to the tropics and subtropics, avocados are a unique fruit and concentrated source of nutrients. The California avocado has a smooth skin, while the Florida avocado (or alligator pear) has a tough and wrinkled exterior. More like a nut than a fruit, these South American natives supply heart-healthy monounsaturated fat and vitamin B_6, magnesium to bolster insulin function, and glutathione for antioxidant protection. Holy guacamole!

❖ **Serving.** One (6 oz) avocado contains 204 calories, 3.8 grams of protein, 13.3 grams of carbohydrate, 17 grams of fat, no cholesterol, and 9.3 grams of dietary fiber. The same serving provides 19 percent of the RDA for vitamin A (186 RE), 15 percent of the RDA for folate (60 mcg), 40 percent of the RDA for vitamin C (24 mg), 8 percent of the RDA for vitamin B_6 (0.13 mg), 30 percent of the RDA for niacin (5.9 mg), 27 percent of the RDA for thiamin (0.4 mg), 26 percent of the RDA for magnesium (104 mg), 22 percent of the RDA for riboflavin (0.4 mg), 11 percent of the RDA for iron (1.6 mg), and 1,484 milligrams of potassium.

❖ **Selecting and storing.** Like many fruits, avocados ripen best off the tree. Ripe avocados yield to gentle palm pressure, but firm, unripe avocados are what are usually found in the market. Select those that are unblemished and heavy for their size. To speed the ripening process, place several avocados in a paper bag and set aside at room temperature for two to four days. Ripe avocados can be stored in the refrigerator several days. Once avocado flesh is cut and exposed to the air, it tends to discolor rapidly, so add lemon or lime juice to help prevent discoloration.

 Kitchen Prescription

Awesome avocados make the base for our Cream of Asparagus Soup that's also full of fiber.

Barley

Beige and shaped like a flattened oval, this grain is usually sold pearled, where it is hulled and polished to cook more quickly. Barley can also be found in quick-cooking, whole-hulled, Job's tears (large hulled grains) grits, flakes, and flour varieties. Hulled or whole-grain barley has only the outer husk removed and is the most nutritious form of the grain. Scotch barley is husked and coarsely ground. Barley grits are hulled barley grains that have been cracked into medium-coarse pieces. It comes in three sizes: coarse, medium, and fine and is good in soups and stews. Used to make beer, whiskey, and cattle feed, barley is a gluten grain and should be avoided by those with gluten sensitivity. Barley provides heart-healthy tocotrienols (a form of vitamin E).

✤ **Serving.** One half cup of cooked pearled barley contains 97 calories, 1.8 grams of protein, 22.3 grams of carbohydrate, 0.4 gram of fat, no cholesterol, and 4.4 grams of dietary fiber. The same serving provides 6 percent of the RDA for folate (12.6 mcg), 8 percent of the RDA for niacin (1.6 mg), and 7 percent of the RDA for iron (1.1 mg).

❖ **Selecting and storing.** Hulled and Scotch barley and barley grits are generally found in health-food stores. Pearl barley has also had the bran removed and has been steamed and polished. Store in an airtight container in a cool, dry place.

 Kitchen Prescription

Opt for hulled barley that still has its germ and bran layers intact, to help keep blood sugar on an even keel.

Beans

Part of the legume family, a good protein source, and a low-glycemic-index food, beans provide a bevy of phytonutrients to benefit diabetes and protect the heart. Filled with phytoestrogens, insoluble fiber, and saponins, these packages of protection are a mainstay in your diet for optimum health.

❖ **Serving.** One half cup of cooked black beans contains 113 calories, 7.6 grams of protein, 20.4 grams of carbohydrate, 0.4 grams of fat, no cholesterol, and 7.5 grams of dietary fiber. The same serving size provides 32 percent of the RDA for folate (64.2 mcg), 13 percent of the RDA for magnesium (51.6 mg), and 270.2 milligrams of potassium.

❖ **Selecting and storing.** Dried beans must usually be soaked in water for several hours or overnight to rehydrate them before cooking. Beans labeled "quick-cooking" have been presoaked and redried before packaging; they require no presoaking and take considerably less time to prepare. The texture of these "quick" beans, however, is not as firm to the bite as regular dried beans. Store dried beans in an airtight container for up to a year.

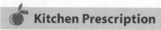

Kitchen Prescription

Try our Bean and Veggie Soup to ladle on the protection.

Blueberries

These berries have been enjoyed by Native Americans and pilgrims and are one of the best-known sources of antioxidants. A true-blue health crusader, blueberries provide anthocyanins that have beneficial effects on fat cells and help to reduce inflammatory cytokines.

❖ **Serving.** One cup of blueberries contains 82 calories, 1 gram of protein, 20.5 grams of carbohydrate, 0.6 gram of fat, no cholesterol, and 3.5 grams of dietary fiber. The same serving provides 315 percent of the RDA for vitamin C (189 mg) and 129 milligrams of potassium.

❖ **Selecting and storing.** Choose blueberries that are firm, uniform in size, and indigo blue with a silvery frost. Discard shriveled or moldy berries. Do not wash until ready to use and store (preferably in a single layer) in a moisture-proof container in the refrigerator for up to five days.

Kitchen Prescription

Get these blue gems in our Berry Tart with Cinnamon Oat Crust.

Broccoli

A descendant of cabbage, broccoli is a member of the cruciferous family of vegetables. Although most broccoli is green, in past times, purple, red, cream, and brown varieties were popular. Broccoli contains lutein to protect the eyes and quercetin, a flavonoid found to help reduce the risk of diabetes.

✤ **Serving.** One half cup of cooked broccoli contains 23 calories, 2.3 grams of protein, 6 grams of carbohydrate, 0.2 gram of fat, no cholesterol, and 2.6 grams of dietary fiber. The same serving provides 11 percent of the RDA for vitamin A (110 RE), 27 percent of the RDA for folate (53.3 mcg), 82 percent of the RDA for vitamin C (49 mg), 10 percent of the RDA for vitamin B_6 (0.2 mg), 6 percent of the RDA for iron (0.9 mg), and 127 milligrams of potassium.

✤ **Selecting and storing.** Look for broccoli with a deep, strong color—green or green with purple. The buds should be tightly closed and the leaves should be crisp. Refrigerate unwashed, in an airtight bag, for up to four days.

Buckwheat

A triangular seed from a fruit relative of rhubarb and sorrel, buckwheat has a nutty flavor and is sold roasted (kasha), whole grain cracked, in unroasted groats grits, or ground into flour. A good source of phytonutrients called sterol, buckwheat may help to reduce cholesterol.

✤ **Serving.** One half cup of cooked buckwheat groats contains 77 calories, 2.8 grams of protein, 16.75 grams of carbohydrate, 0.5 gram of fat, no cholesterol, and 2.7 grams dietary fiber. The same serving provides 7 percent of the RDA for folate (13.9 mcg), 13 percent of the RDA for magnesium (43 mg), and 5 percent of the RDA for iron (0.8 mg).

✤ **Selecting and storing.** Buckwheat groats are the hulled, crushed kernels that are usually cooked in a manner similar to rice. Groats come in coarse, medium, and fine grinds. Kasha, which is roasted buckwheat groats, has a more toasty and nutty flavor. All can be stored in an airtight container in a cool, dry place.

Kitchen Prescription

For more information on how whole grains, such as buckwheat, help to stabilize blood sugar and stave off heart disease, refer back to Chapter 4.

Canola oil

Derived from canola seed and produced in Canada, this oil is minimal in saturated fat. Canola oil provides friendly fats including monounsaturated fat, omega-3 fatty acids, and omega-6 fatty acids

✢ **Serving.** One tablespoon contains 124 calories, no protein, no carbohydrates, 14 grams of fat, 1 gram of saturated fatty acids, 8 grams monounsaturated fat, 4.2 grams polyunsaturated fatty acids, 1.2 grams omega-3s, no cholesterol, and no dietary fiber. The same serving provides 13 percent of the RDA for vitamin E (2.9 mg).

✢ **Selecting and storing.** Store canola oil in a cool, dry place away from sunlight.

Kitchen Prescription

This light oil is perfect for sautéing or using in baked goods. You'll find it in our Tuna Salad with Broccoli, Red Peppers, and Vidalia Onion.

Cantaloupes

This orange-fleshed melon was named after the Italian town of Cantalupa, which also means "wolf howl." The orange color of this juicy melon provides a powerful punch of carotenoids that act as antioxidants and may benefit insulin function.

❖ **Serving.** One half raw cantaloupe (9.5 oz.) contains 95 calories, 2.5 grams of protein, 22.4 grams of carbohydrate, 0.8 gram of fat, no cholesterol, and 2.5 grams of dietary fiber. The same serving provides 86 percent of the RDA for vitamin A (861 RE), 23 percent of the RDA for folate (45.5 mcg), 186 percent of the RDA for vitamin C (112.7 mg), 20 percent of the RDA for vitamin B$_6$ (0.4 mg), and 825 milligrams of potassium.

❖ **Selecting and storing.** Choose cantaloupes that are heavy for their size, have a sweet and fruity fragrance, have a thick and well-raised netting, and yield slightly to pressure at the blossom end. Avoid melons with soft spots or an overly strong odor. Store unripe cantaloupes at room temperature and ripe melons in the refrigerator. Cantaloupes easily absorb other food odors so if you need to refrigerate for more than a day or two, wrap the melon in plastic wrap.

 Kitchen Prescription

Before cutting into these delicious melons, make sure you wash well as bacteria from the outside gets transferred to the inside with the knife blade.

Carrots

As root vegetables that spread from the Middle East to Greece, Rome, and later to Europe, the earliest carrots were not orange, but multicolored. In the 1500s, the carrot showed up in Western Europe, and Dutch cross-breeders developed the modern, orange carrot over the following century. Of course, carrots are full of carotenoids—those antioxidant compounds that help to protect the heart and keep insulin in check.

❖ **Serving.** One medium carrot (2.5 oz.) contains 31 calories, 0.7 gram of protein, 5.6 grams of carbohydrate, 0.1 gram of fat, no cholesterol, and 2 grams of dietary fiber. The same serving provides 202 percent of the RDA for vitamin A (2,025 RE), 5 percent of the RDA for folate (10 mcg), 11 percent of the RDA for vitamin C (6.7 mg), and 233 milligrams of potassium.

❖ **Selecting and storing.** When selecting carrots, choose those that are firm and smooth. Avoid carrots with cracks or any that have begun to soften and wither. Remove carrot greenery as soon as possible because it robs the roots of moisture and vitamins. Store carrots in a plastic bag in the refrigerator's vegetable bin. Avoid storing them near apples, which emit ethylene gas that can give carrots a bitter taste.

Kitchen Prescription

Get Bugs Bunny's favorite food in our Asian Tofu Cakes.

Cherries

Close cousins to the plum, cherries can be sweet or sour, or red or black.

❖ **Serving.** Ten sweet, raw cherries (2.4 oz.) contain 50 calories, 0.9 gram of protein, 11.3 grams of carbohydrate, 0.7 gram of fat, no cholesterol, and 1.5 grams of dietary fiber. The same serving provides 8 percent of the RDA for vitamin C (4.8 mg), 2 percent of the RDA for iron (0.3 mg), and 152 milligrams of potassium.

❖ **Selecting and storing.** Most fresh cherries are available from May (June for sour cherries) through August. Choose brightly colored, shiny, plump cherries. Sweet cherries should be firm, but not hard; sour varieties should be medium firm. Store unwashed cherries in a plastic bag in the refrigerator.

 Kitchen Prescription

Pick cherries for their abundance of flavonoids that help to protect the heart and anthocyanins to help reduce inflammation.

Cranberries

Grown in bogs throughout Asia, Europe, and North America, these berries are best known for a Thanksgiving celebration and their ability to reduce the incidence of bladder infections. These tart treats contain inflammation-reducing anthocyanins.

❖ **Serving.** One cup of raw cranberries contains 46 calories, 0.4 gram of protein, 12.1 grams of carbohydrate, 0.2 gram of fat, no cholesterol, and 4.4 grams of dietary fiber. The same serving provides 21 percent of the RDA for vitamin C (12.8 mg).

❖ **Selecting and storing.** Harvested between Labor Day and Halloween, the peak market period for cranberries is from October through December. They're usually packaged in twelve-ounce plastic bags. Any cranberries that are discolored or shriveled should be discarded. Cranberries can be refrigerated, tightly wrapped, for two months or frozen up to a year.

Kitchen Prescription

Try our Mango and Cranberry Bread Pudding for a delicious dessert full of blood-sugar balancing anthocyanins!

Eggplant

A flowering vegetable native to India, the many varieties of this delicious veggie range in color from rich purple to white, in length from two to twelve inches, and in shape from oblong to round. With terpenes to help reduce cholesterol and purple anthocyanins to reduce inflammation, this giant berry makes a healthy and hearty alternative to meat dishes.

❖ **Serving.** One half cup of cooked eggplant contains 13 calories, 0.4 gram of protein, 3.2 grams of carbohydrate, 0.1 gram of fat, no cholesterol, and 1.2 grams of dietary fiber. The same serving provides 3 percent of the RDA for folate (6.9 mcg) and 119 milligrams of potassium.

❖ **Selecting and storing.** Available year-round, eggplant's peak season is August and September. Choose a firm, smooth-skinned eggplant heavy for its size, and avoid those with soft or brown spots. They should be stored in a cool, dry place and used within a day or two of purchase. If longer storage is necessary, place the eggplant in the refrigerator vegetable drawer.

Kitchen Prescription

Try our Stuffed Eggplant with Peanut Sauce for a meatless meal full of fiber and protein.

Fish

Fish has been the subject of much research over the past twenty years since Danish researchers found a link between fish-eating Eskimos and low rates of heart disease. We now know these sea creatures benefit the heart and help to balance blood sugar thanks to their omega-3 fatty acids.

❖ **Serving.** One serving (3 oz.) of salmon baked or broiled contains 149 calories, 20.5 grams of protein, 0.4 gram of carbohydrate, 6.8 grams of fat, 35.7 milligrams of cholesterol, and no dietary fiber. The same serving provides 122 percent of the RDA for niacin (24.5 mg), 115 percent of the RDA for vitamin B_{12} (2.3 mg), and 20 percent of the RDA for phosphorus (238 mg).

 Kitchen Prescription

Reel Health! Cold-water fish such as tuna, mackerel, herring, and sardines have higher amounts of omega-3s than do their warm-water kin. In fact, a 3½ ounce portion of sardines contains 5.1 grams of omega-3s, while the same portion sizes of Chinook salmon, Atlantic mackerel, and pink salmon contain 3 grams, 2.2 grams, and 1.9 grams respectively. Learn about omega-3s in Chapter 4 and troll our Fish and Seafood recipe section for perfect fish dishes.

Flaxseed

Flaxseed was an ancient culinary staple used as early as 3000 B.C. and touted for its ability to relieve intestinal discomfort by Hippocrates. It has a mild nutty flavor and is often used simply sprinkled over hot dishes such as cooked cereal or stir-frys. This tiny seed provides essential omega-3 fatty acids to help reduce cholesterol and stabilize blood sugar. It is best to consume flax in the ground form because the whole seeds are difficult for our bodies to digest, and therefore we won't reap all of its health benefits.

❖ **Serving.** 2 tablespoons of ground flaxseed contain 80 calories, 3.2 grams of protein, 5.5 grams of fat, and 4.5 grams of dietary fiber.

❖ **Selecting and storing.** Store in the refrigerator or freezer, where it will keep for up to six months.

 Kitchen Prescription

Get the flax! Try it in our Peach Flax Smoothie or grind it up and sprinkle over oatmeal, yogurt, or your other favorite foods.

Garlic

A member of the allium, or onion family, three major types of garlic are available in the United States: the white-skinned, strongly flavored American garlic; the Mexican garlic; and Italian garlic. The Mexican and Italian varieties both have mauve-colored skins and somewhat milder flavors. Elephant garlic (which is not a true garlic but a relative of the leek), is the most mild flavored of the three. Garlic delivers diabetes-beating phytonutrients such as quercetin and cholesterol-lowering sulfides.

❖ **Serving.** One ounce of garlic contains no calories, no protein, no fat, and no carbohydrate. The same serving provides 15 percent of the RDA for vitamin C and vitamin B_6. Garlic contains allicin, diallyl sulfide, ajoene, and quercetin.

❖ **Selecting and storing.** Fresh garlic is available year-round. Purchase firm, plump bulbs with dry skins. Avoid heads with soft or shriveled cloves and those stored in the refrigerated section of the produce department. Store fresh garlic in an open container (away from other foods) in a cool, dark place. Properly stored, unbroken bulbs can be kept for up to eight weeks, though they will begin to dry out toward the end of that time. Once broken from the bulb, individual cloves will keep from three to ten days.

 Kitchen Prescription

Get these cloves of protection in our Vegetarian Paella.

Ginger

A member of the *Zingiberaceae* family that also includes turmeric, most ginger comes from Jamaica, followed by India, Africa, and China. Compounds in ginger called gingerols have been found to improve insulin sensitivity and prevent the oxidation of LDL cholesterol that increases the risk for heart disease.

❖ **Serving.** One tablespoon of grated ginger contains 4 calories, 0.1 gram of protein, 0.9 gram of carbohydrate, 0.1 gram of fat, no cholesterol, and 0.1 gram of dietary fiber. One tablespoon also provides 46 milligrams of potassium.

❖ **Selecting and storing.** Look for ginger with smooth skin and a fresh, spicy fragrance. Fresh unpeeled gingerroot, tightly wrapped, can be refrigerated for up to three weeks and frozen for up to six months.

 Kitchen Prescription

Get your ginger in our Grilled Tuna with Mango Kiwi Salsa or our Sautéed Shrimp and Snow Peas with Rice Noodles.

Grapefruit

A member of the citrus family of fruits grown in Florida, the grapefruit has been purported as a weight-loss aid. Providing heart-helping flavonoids and cholesterol-lowering pectin, grapefruit falls on the low end of the glycemic index scale—making it a great choice to control weight and blood sugar levels.

❖ **Serving.** One half grapefruit contains approximately 45 calories, 1 gram of protein, 12 grams of carbohydrate, 0.1 gram of fat, no cholesterol, and 1.6 grams of dietary fiber. The same serving provides 6 percent of the RDA for folate (11.8 mcg) and 66 percent of the RDA for vitamin C (39.3 mg).

❖ **Selecting and storing.** Fresh grapefruit is available year-round. Those from Arizona and California are in the market from about January through August, while Florida and Texas grapefruits usually arrive around October and last through June. Choose grapefruit that have thin, fine-textured, brightly colored skin. They should be firm yet springy when held in the palm and pressed. Grapefruit keeps best when wrapped in a plastic bag and placed in the vegetable drawer of the refrigerator for up to two weeks.

 Kitchen Prescription

When you choose red grapefruit, you'll also get a dose of heart-protecting lycopene.

Lemons

Citrus fruits cultivated in tropical and temperate climates around the world, lemons add zest and an abundance of vitamin C to foods and beverages. With cholesterol-lowering terpenes and the antioxidant vitamin C, this tangy citrus falls low on the glycemic index.

❖ **Serving.** One tablespoon of lemon juice contains 4 calories, 0.1 gram of protein, 1.4 grams of carbohydrate, no fat, no cholesterol and no dietary fiber. The same serving provides 11 percent of the RDA for vitamin C (75 mg).

❖ **Selecting and storing.** Lemons are available year-round, peaking during the summer months. Choose fruit with smooth, brightly colored skin with no tinge of green. Lemons should be firm, plump, and heavy for their size. Depending on their condition when purchased, they can be refrigerated in a plastic bag for two to three weeks.

 Kitchen Prescription

Have a Boca Cocktail, a favorite refreshment of the Boca Raton, Florida, crowd, to hydrate you through the day and deliver health-promoting phytonutrients. Just squeeze some fresh lemon into your spring water and voila!

Lentils

Members of the legume family, lentils come in red, green, and brown varieties. Phytoestrogens and fiber team up to make these high protein morsels perfect for reducing blood sugar and cholesterol levels.

❖ **Serving.** One half cup cooked lentils contains 101 calories, 7.4 grams of protein, 18.4 grams of carbohydrate, no fat, no cholesterol, and 9 grams of dietary fiber. The same serving provides

86 percent of the RDA for folate (172.7 mcg), 15 percent of the RDA for iron (0.8 mg), and 7 percent of the RDA for thiamin (0.1 mg).

✤ **Selecting and storing.** Lentils should be stored in an airtight container at room temperature and will keep up to a year.

 Kitchen Prescription

Love your legumes! Try our Crunchy Lentil Salad to fill you up without weighing you down!

Mangoes

Cultivated in India for several thousand years, mangoes come in hundreds of varieties. These tropical fruits are high in antioxidants including vitamins C and E, plus carotenoids to help protect the heart and keep insulin in check.

✤ **Serving.** One mango (about 7.3 oz) contains 128 calories, 1 gram of protein, 33.4 grams of carbohydrate, 0.57 gram of fat, no cholesterol, and 3.7 grams of dietary fiber. The same serving provides 77 percent of the RDA for vitamin A (766 RE), 90 percent of the RDA for vitamin C (54 mg), 24 percent of the RDA for vitamin E (2.4 mg), and 14 percent of the RDA for vitamin B$_6$ (0.28 mg).

✤ **Selecting and storing.** Mangoes are in season from May to September, though imported fruit is in the stores sporadically throughout the remainder of the year. Look for fruit with an unblemished, yellow skin blushed with red.

Kitchen Prescription

Try a hot twist on this cool fruit with our Mango and Cranberry Bread Pudding.

Nuts

Scientists speculate nuts may have been around tens of millions of years ago when the continents were still fused—a landmass known as Pangea. We know this because nuts are native to both the Old World and New. Cultivated for twelve thousand years, nuts are one of nature's richest foods. More than three hundred types of nuts exist, but those most commonly enjoyed include almonds, Brazil nuts, cashews, chestnuts, coconuts, hazelnuts, peanuts, pecans, pistachios, walnuts, as well as hickory nuts, pine nuts, and macadamia nuts. Full of minerals and packed with healthy fats, nuts help balance blood sugar and protect the heart by reducing cholesterol.

❖ **Serving.** See labels on individual packages of nuts for serving information.

❖ **Selecting and storing.** Store nuts in closed containers in the refrigerator or freezer to avoid rancidity. It is best to buy fresh raw nuts with shells, as they will store longer than shelled, cooked varieties.

 Kitchen Prescription

Loaded with the "good" fats and minerals, nuts are a great snack and easily incorporated into salads and smoothies. One of the most healthful choice is raw, unblanched almonds.

Oats

A highly rich, protein grain eaten in prepared cereals or as a hot cereal, oats are an American staple. The FDA awarded the first food-specific health claim to oats in January 1997 because of their ability to reduce total and LDL cholesterol. Oats also contain tocotrienol, selenium, beta-glucan, and phytates to help reduce cholesterol and keep blood sugar on an even keel.

✤ **Serving.** One cup of cooked oatmeal (½ cup dry) contains 150 calories, 5.5 grams of protein, 27 grams of carbohydrate, 3 grams of fat, no cholesterol, and 4 grams of dietary fiber. The same serving size provides 13 percent of the RDA for thiamin (0.2 mg), 31 percent of the RDA for magnesium (107 mg), and 9 percent of the RDA for iron (1.9 mg).

✤ **Selecting and storing.** Store oats in a cool, dry place.

 Kitchen Prescription

Get these heart-healthy grains in our Granola recipe.

Olive Oil

Most olive oils come from California but are also imported from France, Greece, Italy, and Spain. They are made by pressing tree-ripened olives to extract a flavorful, heart-healthy monounsaturated oil that is prized throughout the world both for cooking and for salads. The flavor, color, and fragrance of olive oils can vary depending on distinctions such as growing region and the crop's condition. Olive oil also contains phenols.

❖ **Serving.** One tablespoon of extra-virgin olive oil contains 120 calories, no protein, no carbohydrates, 14 grams of fat, no cholesterol, and no dietary fiber.

❖ **Selecting and storing.** Olive oil should be stored in a cool, dark place and will keep for up to six months. It can be refrigerated, in which case it will last up to a year.

 Kitchen Prescription

All olive oils are graded in accordance with the degree of acidity they contain. The best are cold-pressed, a chemical-free process that involves only pressure, which produces a natural level of low acidity. Extra-virgin olive oil (the cold-pressed) is a result of the first pressing of the olives, and contains only 1 percent of acid. It is considered the finest and fruitiest of the olive oils and is therefore also the most expensive. It can range from a champagne color to greenish-golden to bright green. In general, the deeper the color, the more intense the olive flavor and more phytonutrients present.

Onions

Members of the allium family, onions have two main classifications: green and dry. Dry onions are simply mature onions with a juicy flesh covered with dry, papery skin. With their cholesterol-reducing sulfur compounds and diabetes-beating quercetin, onions add flavor and health to any dish.

❖ **Serving.** One medium, raw onion contains 60 calories, 2 grams of protein, 14 grams of carbohydrate, no fat, no cholesterol, and 3 grams of dietary fiber. The same serving also provides 18 percent of the RDA for vitamin C (12 mg).

❖ **Selecting and storing.** When buying onions, choose those that are heavy for their size with dry, papery skins and no signs of spotting or moistness. Avoid onions with soft spots. Store in a cool, dry place with good air circulation. Depending on their condition when purchased, onions will keep for up to two months. Once cut, an onion should be tightly wrapped, refrigerated, and used within four days.

 Kitchen Prescription

Toss them into salads, dice and sauté into sauces, or chop and add them to soups.

Oranges

The most popular citrus fruit, oranges are believed to have originated in Southeast Asia and were brought to the New World by Christopher Columbus. A low-GI food, oranges also provide flavonoids, carotenoids, terpenes, pectin, and glutathione. Refer back to Chapter 5 for how these citrus phytonutrients can fight diabetes and protect the heart.

❖ **Serving.** One orange (approximately 4.6 oz.) contains 62 calories, 1.3 grams of protein, 15.4 grams of carbohydrate, 0.2 grams of fat, no cholesterol, and 3 grams of dietary fiber. The same serving provides 20 percent of the RDA for folate (39.7 mcg), 92 percent of the RDA for vitamin C (69.7 mg), 13 percent of the RDA for thiamin (0.2 mg), 4 percent of the RDA for calcium (52 mg), and 237 milligrams of potassium.

❖ **Selecting and storing.** Fresh oranges are available year-round at different times, depending on the variety. Choose fruit that is firm and heavy for its size, with no mold or spongy spots. Oranges can be stored at cool room temperature for a day or so, but should then be refrigerated and should keep for up to two weeks.

Kitchen Prescription

Oranges are an excellent source of vitamin C and carotenoids. Try our Chicken and Orange Stir-Fry with Rice Noodles to get this citrus with a sunny disposition.

Peaches

Widely planted across the eastern seaboard by the early settlers, many botanists thought the fruit to be indigenous to the United States. The peach is the third most popular of all fruits grown in the United States and comes in numerous varieties. With their flavonoids and carotenoids, peaches are sweet on the heart and on the palette.

❖ **Serving.** One peach (approximately 4 oz.) contains 37 calories, 0.7 gram of protein, 9.7 grams of carbohydrate, 0.1 gram of fat, no cholesterol, and 1.5 grams of dietary fiber. The same serving also provides 47 percent of the RDA for vitamin A (465 RE), 19 percent of the RDA for vitamin C (1.7 mg), and 8 percent of the RDA for niacin (1.5 mg).

❖ **Selecting and storing.** Peaches are available from May to October in most regions of the United States. Look for fragrant fruit that gives slightly to palm pressure. Avoid those with signs of greening.

 Kitchen Prescription

Whether ripe off the tree or enjoyed in our Peach Flax Smoothie, these fuzzy fruits pack a powerful phytonutrient punch.

Peppers

Thought by the Europeans in the 1600s to cure digestive problems and ulcers, modern medicine has shown that peppers contain numerous compounds that have beneficial effects on the digestive system. Many varieties of peppers exist, including banana peppers, red bell, yellow bell, green bell, chili, cayenne, jalapeño, habanero, and Scotch bonnet. Along with vitamin C and magnesium, if you choose red peppers you'll also get a dose of lycopene.

✤ **Serving.** One half cup of red bell pepper contains 14 calories, 0.5 gram of protein, 3.2 grams of carbohydrate, 0.1 gram of fat, no cholesterol, and 1.8 grams of dietary fiber. The same serving also provides 11 percent of the RDA for folate (22.2 mcg), 44 percent of the RDA for vitamin C (26.1 mg), 35 percent of the RDA for vitamin B_6 (0.7 mg), 17 percent of the RDA for niacin (3.3 mg), 18 percent of the RDA for thiamin (0.2 mg), 14 percent of the RDA for magnesium (54.5 mg), 19 percent of the RDA for iron (2.8 mg), and 844 milligrams of potassium.

✤ **Selecting and storing.** Choose peppers that are firm; have a brightly colored, shiny skin; and are heavy for their size. Avoid peppers that are limp, shriveled, or have soft or bruised spots. Store peppers in a plastic bag in the refrigerator for up to a week.

 Kitchen Prescription

Pick a peck in our Chicken Jambalaya. You can substitute red peppers for green to get your lycopene.

Pomegranates

An unusual fruit with bright red juice and many seeds, the name *pomegranate* comes from two French words, *pome* and *granate* literally meaning "apple with many seeds." These unique fruits provide a good dose of fiber plus anthocyanins to help reduce inflammatory cytokines.

❖ **Serving.** One pomegranate (approximately 5.5 oz.) contains 104 calories, 1.5 grams of protein, 26.5 grams of carbohydrate, 0.5 gram of fat, no cholesterol, and 1 gram of dietary fiber. The same serving also provides 16 percent of the RDA for vitamin C (9.4 mg) and 399 milligrams of potassium.

❖ **Selecting and storing.** In the United States pomegranates are available in October and November. Choose those that are heavy for their size and have a bright, fresh color and blemish-free skin. Refrigerate for up to two months or store in a cool, dark place for up to a month.

 Kitchen Prescription

Sprinkle pomegranate buds onto a salad or on top of your favorite cereal in the morning!

Pumpkins

A flowering vegetable and members of the gourd family, pumpkins are powerhouses of carotenoids to be enjoyed year-round.

❖ **Serving.** One half cup of canned pumpkin contains 41 calories, 1.3 grams of protein, 9.9 grams of carbohydrate, 0.3 gram of fat, no cholesterol, and 3.6 grams of dietary fiber. The same serving also provides 269 percent of the RDA for vitamin A

(2,691 RE), 8 percent of the RDA for folate (15 mcg), 9 percent of the RDA for vitamin C (5.1 mg), 11 percent of the RDA for iron (1.7 mg), 7 percent of the RDA for magnesium (28 mg), and 251 milligrams of potassium.

❖ **Selecting and storing.** Fresh pumpkins are available in the fall and winter and some specimens have weighed in at well over one hundred pounds. In general, however, the flesh from smaller sizes will be more tender and succulent. Choose pumpkins that are free from blemishes and heavy for their size. Store whole pumpkins at room temperature up to a month or refrigerate up to three months.

 Kitchen Prescription

Get your carotenoids and fiber from our Tahinos Pumpkin Chowder.

Raspberries

Typically red, raspberries also come in other colors such as purple, yellow, amber, and black. These antioxidant-rich berries provide flavonoids and vitamin C.

❖ **Serving.** One cup of raspberries contains 61 calories, 1.2 grams of protein, 14.3 grams of carbohydrates, 0.7 gram of fat, no cholesterol, and 8 grams of dietary fiber. The same serving provides 16 percent of the RDA for folate (32 mcg), 51 percent of the RDA for vitamin C (30.8 mg), 6 percent of the RDA for magnesium (22 mg), and 5 percent of the RDA for iron (0.7 mg).

❖ **Selecting and storing.** Raspberries are available from May through November. Choose brightly colored, plump berries without the hull. If the hulls are still attached, the berries were picked too early and will undoubtedly be tart. Avoid soft, shriveled, or moldy berries. Store in a dry container in the refrigerator for two to three days. If necessary, rinse lightly just before serving.

Kitchen Prescription

Chocolate and raspberries come together in our Chocolate Mint Berry Smoothie for a healthy delight filled with phytonutrients!

Rice

Originating from Southeast Asia, rice is the second most consumed food in the world. Enjoy whole-grain brown rice with its B vitamins, including B$_6$, which reduces levels of heart-harming homocysteine, and magnesium, important for insulin function.

❖ **Serving.** One half cup of cooked medium-grain brown rice contains 110 calories, 2.3 grams of protein, 23 grams of carbohydrate, 0.8 gram of fat, no cholesterol, and 1.7 grams of dietary fiber. The same serving provides 10 percent of the RDA for vitamin B$_6$ (0.2 mg), 5 percent of the RDA for niacin (1 mg), 67 percent of the RDA for thiamin (1 mg), 11 percent of the RDA for magnesium (43 mg), and 3 percent of the RDA for iron (0.5 mg).

❖ **Selecting and storing.** Because of the presence of the bran, brown rice is subject to rancidity, which limits its shelf life to only about six months.

Kitchen Prescription

Don't forget to keep those germ and bran layers on! Buy unrefined brown rice to keep your blood sugar on an even keel.

Soybeans

Members of the legume family, and a complete protein, soybeans
are a main staple of the Asian diet. Soybeans provide phytoestrogens, isoflavones, and saponins to keep blood sugar in check
and reduce cholesterol.

✤ **Serving.** One quarter block of tofu (approximately 4 oz.)
contains 90 calories, 9.4 grams of protein, 2.2 grams of carbohydrate, 5.4 grams of fat, no cholesterol, and 1.4 grams of dietary
fiber. The same serving provides 30 percent of the RDA for magnesium (120 mg), 41 percent of the RDA for iron (6.2 mg), and
10 percent of the RDA for calcium (122 mg).

✤ **Selecting and storing.** Tofu is very perishable and should be
refrigerated for no more than a week. If it's packaged in water,
drain it, cover with fresh water, and change the water daily. Tofu
can be frozen for up to three months.

 Kitchen Prescription

Try our Spicy Noodles Salad with Baked Tofu for a delicious dose of
phytonutrients with Asian appeal.

Spinach

A leafy, green native of Asia, spinach was brought to Europe by
the Moors when they conquered Spain in the eighth century.
Spinach also contains carotenoids, zeaxanthin, and lutein—to
protect the eyes.

✤ **Serving.** One half cup of cooked spinach contains 21 calories, 2.7 grams of protein, 3.4 grams of carbohydrate, 0.2 gram
of fat, no cholesterol, and 2.1 grams of dietary fiber. The same

serving provides 74 percent of the RDA for vitamin A (737 RE), 66 percent of the RDA for folate (131.2 mcg), 20 percent of the RDA for magnesium (78.3 mg), 21 percent of the RDA for iron (3.2 mg), and 10 percent of the RDA for calcium (122.4 mg).

✤ **Selecting and storing.** Fresh spinach is available year-round. Choose leaves that are crisp and dark green with a nice fresh fragrance. Avoid those that are limp, damaged, or have yellow spots. Refrigerate in a plastic bag for up to three days.

 Kitchen Prescription

Spinach, which is usually very gritty, must be thoroughly rinsed. Get it in our Vegetable Frittata, our Mediterranean Spinach Pie, or our Spinach Salad with Figs, Red Onion, and Goat Cheese.

Strawberries

The most popular American berry, more than seventy varieties of this nutrient-rich food exist. With their red color, these boisterous berries boast lycopene as one phytonutrient in their disease-fighting arsenal.

✤ **Serving.** One cup of raw strawberries contains 45 calories, 1 gram of protein, 10.5 grams of carbohydrate, 0.6 gram of fat, no cholesterol, and 2.9 grams of dietary fiber. The same serving provides 13 percent of the RDA for folate (26.4 mcg), 141 percent of the RDA for vitamin C (84.5 mg), 4 percent of the RDA for iron (0.6 mg), and 247 milligrams of potassium.

✤ **Selecting and storing.** Fresh strawberries are available year-round in many regions of the country, with the peak season from April to June. Choose brightly colored, plump berries that still have their leaves attached. Avoid soft, shriveled, or moldy berries.

Do not wash until ready to use, and store in a dry container in the refrigerator for two to three days.

Kitchen Prescription

Give it a whirl and try our Strawberry Banana Smoothie. As bananas are high on the glycemic index, have it as a post-workout treat.

Tea

Used by the ancient Chinese, the Greeks, medieval herbalists, and scholars of the enlightenment for their medicinal purposes, black tea, green tea, and oolong tea come from the *Camellia sinensis* plant. Phytonutrients in tea, such as catechins and tannins, help to balance blood sugar. So get out the kettle!

❖ **Serving.** Six ounces of black tea contains 2 calories, no protein, 0.5 gram of carbohydrate, no fat, no cholesterol, and no dietary fiber. The same serving provides 5 percent of the RDA for folate (1 mcg).

❖ **Selecting and storing.** Store tea bags or loose tea in an airtight container in a cool dry place.

Kitchen Prescription

Try our Spiced Chai or Gingered Green Tea Cooler. If you're pressed for time, try Tazo's Chai or Tazo's Zen.

Tomatoes

Thought to have originated from South America, tomatoes were transported by Spanish explorers to Europe in the 1500s. Most notable for their lycopene, tomatoes help to protect the heart by reducing oxidation of LDL cholesterol.

❖ **Serving.** One red ripe tomato (approximately 4.3 oz.) contains 24 calories, 1.1 grams of protein, 5.3 grams of carbohydrate, 0.3 gram of fat, no cholesterol, and 1.3 grams dietary fiber. The same serving provides 14 percent of the RDA for vitamin A (139 RE), 6 percent of the RDA for folate (11.6 mcg), 36 percent of the RDA for vitamin C (21.6 mg), and 5 percent of the RDA for iron (0.8 mg).

❖ **Selecting and storing.** Choose firm, well-shaped tomatoes that are fragrant and richly colored (for their variety). They should be free from blemishes, heavy for their size, and give slightly to pressure. Ripe tomatoes should be stored at room temperature and used within a few days, as cold temperatures make the flesh pithy.

 Kitchen Prescription

Cooking tomatoes helps to unlock lycopene, a fat-soluble nutrient. Adding a bit of oil also helps aid in the absorption. So get out the saucepan!

Wheat

One of the oldest grains cultivated, wheat is available in numerous forms including wheat berries, cracked wheat, bulgur grits, shredded wheat, unprocessed bran (or miller's bran), wheat germ, rolled wheat flakes, puffed wheat, cream of wheat, and wheat flour.

❖ **Serving.** One slice of whole-wheat bread contains 90 calories, 4 grams of protein, 15 grams of carbohydrate, 1 gram of fat, no cholesterol, and 3 grams of dietary fiber. The same serving provides 2 percent of the RDA for folate (4.1 mcg), 6 percent of the RDA for niacin (1.2 mg), 6 percent of the RDA for thiamin (0.09 mg), and 2 percent of the RDA for riboflavin (0.04 mg).

❖ **Selecting and storing.** Whole-wheat flour contains part of the grain's germ and turns rancid quickly because of the oil in the germ. Refrigerate or freeze these flours tightly wrapped and use as soon as possible.

 Kitchen Prescription

Don't forget to look for the words *whole grain* when buying wheat. Whole-grain products have not been refined or stripped of their nutritious germ and bran layers, which help to stabilize blood sugar.

So far we've examined the various nutritional elements in different foods and diets. Next, you'll learn which herbs and spices you should be stocking in your kitchen.

Healing Herbs and Spices

THE FRAGRANT SMELL of spiced chai doesn't just lend flavor but also an abundance of blood-sugar balancing compounds. We are beginning to understand that our spice rack and herb garden don't just please the palette but are packed with—what else?—phytonutrients! Researchers at the Cytokine Research Laboratory, Department of Experimental Therapeutics at the University of Texas uniquely describe this as the "reasoning for seasoning." This chapter illustrates some of the diabetes-beating herbs and spices, the phytonutrients responsible for their delicious protection, and how to use them with the recipes from Chapter 10 to create meals that heal!

Savoring Flavor

For centuries, these flavor boosters have been used to jazz up cuisine, as well as treat illnesses and prevent spoilage. In ancient times, people prized spices more highly than gold or jewels. In today's world of high-sodium and high-fat processed foods, savvy consumers are turning to herbs and spices to add flavor and zest to their meals. Nature's flavor enhancers deliver an abundance of sugar balancers and heart protectors while eliminating added calories and salt.

A Spice Rack for Diabetes Protection

Unlike herbs, which come from the leaves of plants, spices are made from the buds, barks, fruits, seeds, or roots. Although research of the healing powers of spices is relatively new, scientists' discoveries thus far have been impressive. Let's find out how a dash can put a damper on diabetes and reduce the risk for heart disease.

Kitchen Prescription

Boost the flavor of spices by toasting them briefly in a dry skillet until slightly brown and aromatic

Allspice. This is the dried, unripe berry of *Pimenta dioica*, an evergreen tree in the myrtle family. After drying, the berries are small, dark brown balls just a little larger than peppercorns. Allspice comes from Jamaica, Mexico, and Honduras. Pungent and fragrant, it is not a blend of "all spices," but its taste and aroma remind many people of a mix of cloves, cinnamon, and nutmeg. Allspice contains numerous health-promoting phytonutrients that have insulin-like activity and may help to reduce blood sugar.

Kitchen Prescription

Allspice is used in Jamaican jerk seasoning and in Jamaican soups, stews, and curries. It also is used in pickling spice, spiced tea mixes, cakes, cookies and pies.

Anise. The anise seed is a gray-brown oval seed from *Pimpinella anisum*, a plant in the Umbelliferae, or carrot, family. It is related to caraway, dill, cumin, and fennel. Spain and Mexico are the sources for anise, although it is native to the Middle East. Anise, which smells and tastes like licorice, contains phytonutrients called terpenoids that have been found to help to reduce cholesterol.

 Kitchen Prescription

You can use anise in cakes, cookies, and sweet breads, like Europeans do, or in soups and stews, as is done in the Middle East and India.

Bay Leaves. Grown in the Mediterranean region and a staple in most American kitchens, bay leaves contain numerous health-promoting phytonutrients that have insulin-like activity and may help to reduce blood sugar. They come from the sweet bay or laurel tree, known botanically as *Laurus nobilis*. The elliptical leaves of both trees are green, glossy, and grow up to three inches long. Bay leaves can be used in soups, stews, or meat and vegetable dishes. The leaves also flavor classic French dishes such as bouillabaisse.

 Kitchen Prescription

Try it in our Bean and Veggie Soup for a dish full of fiber.

Cinnamon. Cinnamon is the dried bark of various laurel trees in the cinnamomum family. The cinnamon used in North America is from the cassia tree, which is grown in Vietnam, China, Indonesia, and Central America. Available in both ground and stick forms, cinnamon has a sweet, woody fragrance that enhances the taste of vegetables and fruits. It contains phytonutrients called polyphenols that may help reduce blood sugar and protect the heart. A recent study showed that regular consumption of as little as 1 gram of cinnamon is beneficial for those with elevated glucose, triglyceride, or LDL or total cholesterol and helps reduce the risk of cardiovascular disease associated with diabetes.

 Kitchen Prescription

Get your dose of cinnamon in our Spiced Chai.

Cloves. These are the rich, brown, dried, unopened flower buds of *Syzygium aromaticum*, an evergreen tree in the myrtle family. The name comes from the French *clou* meaning nail. Cloves come from Madagascar, Brazil, Panang, and Ceylon and are strong, pungent, and sweet. Cloves contain a phytonutrient called *eugenol* that has insulin-like activity and helps to reduce blood sugar.

 Kitchen Prescription

Try cloves in our Chicken Jambalaya for some spicy protection.

Cumin. This is the pale green seed of *Cuminum cyminum*, a small herb in the Umbelliferae or carrot family. The cumin seed is uniformly elliptical, deeply furrowed, and frequently used in Mexican dishes. It has a distinctive, slightly bitter yet warm flavor. Cumin contains numerous phytonutrients including thymoquinone that helps to reduce cholesterol and triglycerides, as well as reduce inflammation.

 Kitchen Prescription

Get it in our Turkey, Avocado, and Tomato Tostadas.

Fennel. This seed is the oval, green or yellowish-brown dried fruit of *Foeniculum vulgare*, a member of the Umbelliferae or carrot family. Fennel has an aniselike flavor but is more aromatic, sweeter, and less pungent. Fennel contains phytonutrients including *terpenoids* that help to reduce cholesterol and inflammation.

 Kitchen Prescription

Fennel goes well with fish and is used in some curry powder mixes.

Ginger. A member of the Zingiberaceae family—which includes turmeric—ginger comes mainly from Jamaica, India, Africa, and China. With a peppery and slightly sweet flavor and a spicy and pungent aroma, this extremely versatile root has long been a mainstay in Asian and Indian cooking and found its way early on into European foods as well. Young ginger, often called spring ginger, has a pale, thin skin that requires no peeling. Mature ginger has a tough skin that must be peeled away to preserve the delicate flesh just under the surface. Ginger contains phytonutrients, like *zingibain*, and *gingerols* that help to enhance insulin sensitivity. This root has also been found to protect the heart by reducing the stickiness of platelets and preventing the oxidation of LDL cholesterol.

 Kitchen Prescription

Get zingy ginger in our Gingered Green Tea Cooler for a Zen feel with health appeal!

Saffron. In its pure form, saffron is a mass of compressed, threadlike, dark orange strands. The stigma of *Crocus sativus*, a flowering plant in the crocus family, saffron is native to the

Mediterranean. The world's most expensive spice, more than 225,000 stigmas must be handpicked to produce one pound. Primarily cultivated in Spain, saffron is used in French bouillabaisse, Spanish paella, and many Middle Eastern dishes. Saffron has a spicy, pungent, and bitter flavor with a sharp and penetrating odor. It contains a phytonutrient called *crocin* that has more antioxidant punch than vitamin E (alpha-tocopherol). It also helps to reduce the oxidation of cholesterol, a key factor in the development of heart disease.

 Kitchen Prescription

Try this pricey spice in our Steamed Mussels with Saffron Sauce.

Turmeric. From the root of *Curcuma longa*, a leafy plant in the Zingiberaceae or ginger family, this root, or rhizome, has a tough brown skin and bright orange flesh. Ground turmeric comes from fingers that extend from the root. It is boiled or steamed and then dried and ground. India is the world's primary producer of turmeric, but it is also grown in China and Indonesia. It is mildly aromatic, has scents of orange or ginger, and has a pungent, bitter flavor. Turmeric contains a powerful phytonutrient called *curcumin*. Studies show that turmeric may help to reduce blood sugar and protect the kidneys by reducing blood cholesterol levels.

 Kitchen Prescription

Turmeric is a necessary ingredient of curry powder and is used extensively in Indian dishes, including lentil and meat dishes, and in Southeast Asian cooking. Try this golden spice in our Vegetable Frittata.

Herbs for Health

Prior to the discovery of modern pharmaceuticals, healers relied on herbs to treat illness and promote health. Researchers now know that the phytonutrients in herbs provide a range of health benefits from reducing cholesterol, preventing cancer, easing menopausal symptoms, and more. Although numerous healing herbs exist, we will focus on some of the most common culinary herbs that bring aroma to your kitchen and an added dose of health to your meals.

Basil. A bright green, leafy plant, *Ocimum basilicum*, basil is in the Labitae or mint family. Grown primarily in the United States, France, and the Mediterranean region, basil is widely used in Italian cuisine and is often paired with tomatoes. It is also used in Thai cooking. Basil has a sweet, herbal bouquet and its name means "be fragrant." Compounds in basil, including terpenoids and *rosmarinic acid*, help to reduce cholesterol and may also help to lower blood sugar.

 Kitchen Prescription

Get a delicious dose of basil in our Tuna Salad with Broccoli, Red Peppers, and Vidalia.

Cilantro. This is the leaf of the young coriander plant, *Coriandrum sativum*, an herb in the Umbelliferae or carrot family, similar to anise. Grown in California and traditionally used in Middle Eastern, Mexican, and Asian cooking, cilantro's taste is a fragrant mix of parsley and citrus. Cilantro contains phytonutrients that may help to reduce cholesterol and triglycerides levels by breaking down lipids. In fact, cilantro's cholesterol-reducing effects were comparable with that of the cholesterol-lowering drug Liponil in a recent study.

Kitchen Prescription

Try cilantro in our Chicken Tomatillo Enchilada.

Dill. A tall, feathery annual, *Anethum graveolens*, dill is in the Umbelliferae or carrot family. Both dill seed and weed (dried leaves) come from the same plant and are widely used in pickling as well as in German, Russian, and Scandinavian dishes. The dill seed flavor is clean, pungent, and reminiscent of caraway; dill weed has a similar but mellower and fresher flavor. Dill contains phytonutrients including *myristicin* and *apiol*, and animal studies have shown that dill may help to reduce triglycerides.

Kitchen Prescription

Get a dose of dill in our Dilled Chicken Salad Wrap.

Marjoram. Marjoram is the gray-green leaf of *Majorana hortensis*, a low-growing member of the Labitae or mint family. Often mistaken for oregano, marjoram has a delicate, sweet, pleasant flavor with a slightly bitter undertone. As a member of the mint family, marjoram contains numerous antioxidant compounds including terpenes that may help to reduce cholesterol.

Kitchen Prescription

Get marjoram in our Crunchy Lentil Salad that is full of fiber.

Mint. This is the dried leaf of a perennial herb in the Labitae family. There are two important species, *Mentha spicata L.* (spearmint) and *Mentha piperita L.* (peppermint). It is strong and sweet with a tangy flavor and a cool aftertaste. Antioxidant compounds in mint, including terpenoids, have been found to reduce total and LDL cholesterol, reducing the risk for heart disease.

 Kitchen Prescription

Try our Chocolate Mint Berry Smoothie for a mouth-watering medley.

Oregano. Mediterranean oregano is the dried leaf of *Origanum vulgare L.*, a perennial herb in the Labitae or mint family. Mexican oregano is the dried leaf of one of several plants of the Lippia genus. Grown in California and New Mexico, as well as the Mediterranean region, oregano is the spice that gives pizza its characteristic flavor. It is also usually used in chili powder. Oregano has a pungent odor and flavor with the Mexican variety being a bit stronger than Mediterranean oregano. Studies show that oregano, through its antioxidant phytonutrients like *thymol* and *limonene*, helps to keep blood sugar under control.

 Kitchen Prescription

Try oregano in our Spanish Rice and Chicken Casserole.

Parsley. This is a member of the Umbelliferae or carrot family and is commonly used as a flavoring and garnish. Although more than thirty varieties of this herb exist, the most popular are curly-leaf parsley and the more strongly flavored Italian or flat-leaf parsley. Parsley contains phytonutrients, including *polyacetylenes* and *monoterpenes*, that act as antioxidants and may help to reduce cholesterol. Culinary caution: parsley should not be consumed in large amounts by pregnant women.

 Kitchen Prescription

Get parsley in our Vegetarian Paella.

Rosemary. This herb is in the Labitae or mint family. A small evergreen shrub, native to the Mediterranean, the leaves of *Rosmarinus officinalis* resemble curved pine needles. Rosemary contains rosmarinic acid, among other phytonutrients that help to reduce inflammatory factors involved with the development of heart disease and other chronic illnesses. Rosemary is one of the commonly used herbs that provide substantial amounts of flavonoids, which enhance vitamin C's action. Flavorful flavonoids act as antioxidants, protect LDL cholesterol from oxidation, and reduce the risk for a dangerous clot.

 Kitchen Prescription

Today rosemary is widely produced in France, Spain, and Portugal and has a distinct tealike aroma and a piney flavor.

Sage. This herb is from the evergreen shrub *Salvia officinalis*, in the Labitae or mint family. Grown primarily in the United States as well as Dalmatia and Albania, sage has a fragrant aroma and an astringent but warm flavor. The name *sage* comes from the Latin word *salia*, meaning "to save." Along with a good amount of flavonoids that protect the heart, sage also contains chromium and vitamin C, which have antidiabetic activity.

Kitchen Prescription

Sage's long, grayish-green leaves take on a velvety, cottonlike texture when rubbed (meaning ground lightly and passed through a coarse sieve).

Thyme. Thyme is the leaf of a low-growing shrub called *Thymus vulgaris* in the Labitae or mint family. Its tiny grayish-green leaves rarely are greater than one-fourth of an inch long. For use as a condiment, thyme leaves are dried then chopped or ground. Grown in southern Europe, including France, Spain, and Portugal, thyme is also indigenous to the Mediterranean. Thyme has a subtle, dry aroma and a slightly minty flavor. As part of the mint family, thyme contains compounds that may help to reduce cholesterol, and flavonoids to protect the heart.

Kitchen Prescription

Take the time to try thyme in our Risotto Tart with Tomatoes, Onions, and Peppers.

Perfect Pairings

Now that we have explored some of the healing properties of herbs and spices, let's take a look at the flavor combinations that please the palette. Don't be afraid to experiment and create your own blends to design savory and healthy meals.

* **Poultry:** rosemary and thyme; tarragon, marjoram, and garlic; cumin, bay leaf, and saffron (or turmeric); ginger, cinnamon, and allspice; curry powder and thyme

* **Fish and seafood:** cumin and oregano; tarragon, thyme, parsley, and garlic; thyme, fennel, saffron, and red pepper; ginger, sesame, and white pepper; cilantro, parsley, cumin, and garlic
* **Beans:** marjoram and rosemary, caraway and dry mustard
* **Broccoli:** ginger and garlic, sesame and nutmeg
* **Cabbage:** celery seeds and dill, curry powder and nutmeg
* **Carrots:** cinnamon and nutmeg, ginger
* **Corn:** chili powder and cumin, dill
* **Peas:** anise, rosemary and marjoram
* **Spinach:** curry powder and ginger, nutmeg and garlic
* **Summer squash:** mint and parsley, tarragon and garlic
* **Winter squash:** cinnamon and nutmeg, allspice and red pepper
* **Tomatoes:** basil and rosemary, cinnamon and ginger
* **Potatoes:** dill and parsley, caraway, nutmeg and chives
* **Rice:** chili powder and cumin; curry powder, ginger, and coriander; cinnamon, cardamom, and cloves
* **Pasta:** basil, rosemary, and parsley; cumin, turmeric, and red pepper; oregano and thyme

Along with building your spice rack with healing herbs and spices, in the next chapter, we offer tips for other items to put into your shopping cart to prevent and manage diabetes.

8

Shopping for Health

CHOOSING THE RIGHT ingredients is the first step to eating healthier to manage or prevent diabetes. Unfortunately, with so many products on the market, selecting healthful items to stock your pantry can be a daunting task. In this chapter, we give you practical tips on deciphering food labels and the art of shopping for health.

Strategies for Smart Shopping

Understanding the science behind how foods can protect us is only useful when we can translate that information into our grocery carts and ultimately onto our tables. Because most of us spend a substantial amount of time at the grocery (84 percent of consumers prepare home-cooked meals at least three times a week), it is critical to navigate the supermarket smorgasbord to find the healthiest products.

Proper Planning for Healthy Choices

Proper planning helps to deter those dinky Twinkies from jumping in your cart and wrecking your health. Here are a few practical tips to keep you in line at the store.

Before you go to the store, make a list and check it twice. Smart shopping begins before you leave the house. Being unprepared leads to multiple trips and unwanted, often unhealthy, items finding their way into your shopping cart. Instead of buying on impulse, stray from your list only when the item is a healthy one. If a junior shopper vying for the candy aisle accompanies you, have her explore the produce section and let her choose a unique fruit or vegetable to try (e.g., a persimmon, pomegranate, or kiwi) to foster good health habits.

Also, before you venture to the grocery store, you should eat first. Shopping while hungry is a surefire way to end up straying from your list and succumbing to unhealthy choices. Having a small snack will help you avoid temptations that will wind up in your cupboard and on your waist.

What to Look For

Become a perimeter shopper. The exterior of the store contains many of the whole foods we have described for optimum health. Spend most of your time shopping for fresh produce, seafood, lean meats, and dairy. When choosing dairy, opt for lower calorie products such as shredded mozzarella; fresh, soft cheeses; and yogurt as opposed to aged, hard cheeses like cheddar—which rack up 100 calories for each one-ounce cube.

There is so much variation in the health value of different brands of foods, so pause, read labels, and compare choices. Read ingredient lists; look at calories and sugar, the type of grain used (whole grains versus refined), and the type of oils used (partially hydrogenated palm kernel oil versus olive oil). We will demystify the food label later in this chapter.

Filling Your Cart

It's easy to incorporate all the diabetes-beating foods, herbs, spices plus the "good" fats and "good" carbs we talked about in earlier chapters. Here are some quick tips on stocking your pantry.

Remember those colors we described in Chapter 6? You want to look for those same colors to put them in your cart and build your meals around them. When you look in your shopping cart, the vast majority of your food selection should be fruits and vegetables to reach the goal of at least five to nine servings a day. Blue blueberry smoothies, hearty red marinara sauces, green salads, and multicolor vegetable soups should be your mainstays.

Frozen vegetables, fruits and seafood, and poultry are an economical and convenient way to eat healthy. Having a freezer stocked with these staples ensures you can whip up a delicious meal in minutes. Try frozen fruits like blueberries, mixed berries, or cherries for the smoothies and fruit-based desserts you'll find in Chapter 10. Opt for frozen edamame (soy beans in their pods) for an easy appetizer for an Asian meal. Bagged, mixed veggies are perfect to make vegetable soups like our Bean and Veggie Soup, and research shows that the nutrient content is equal to or greater than fresh foods, which can lose many vitamins in the shipping and handling. By adding a few additional ingredients, frozen foods can provide you with a healthy base for many of your meals.

As we mentioned in Chapter 7, the condiment aisle is full of flavor and a great way to add zesty phytonutrient protection to your meals. Go back to that chapter and make sure you have the right herbs and spices in your kitchen. In addition, purchase high-quality cooking oils like extra-virgin olive oil, sesame oil, canola oil, and other liquid vegetable oils for sautéing or making dressings and marinades. Buy mustard, vinegars, horseradish, and the dried herbs and spices that help prevent and manage diabetes and add virtually no calories and lots of flavor to all varieties of foods.

Finally, go nuts for your health! Instead of chips, pretzels, and other nutrient-void snack foods, opt for raw nuts and seeds, which are full of minerals, good-quality fats, and other health-promoting nutrients. Just be sure to watch your portion size: a quarter cup of almonds, for example, contains 170 calories.

Buyer Beware

Beware of not-so-healthy "health" foods. Sports drinks and energy bars are not much more than sugar fortified with vitamins and minerals, each packing a whopping 200 plus calories per serving. The same goes for desserts and snack foods that are labeled "organic." These are no better than their "conventional" counterparts when it comes to nutrition.

Remember how we talked about the dangers of processed meats and red meats and their effects on diabetes in Chapter 4? That's why it's a good idea to avoid the deli when shopping. Although many deli foods are marketed as "fresh," most are processed red meats or poultry.

Finally, don't drown in the beverage aisle. Other than good old H_2O, there's nothing in the beverage aisle you want to buy. This also goes for sugary, high-calorie iced teas, pseudo-smoothies, sweetened milks, and coffee beverages. Our body doesn't register liquid calories as it does calories from solid foods, which leads to weight gain. Don't be deterred by teas, though, which provide a spectrum of antioxidant phytonutrients and help to balance blood sugar.

Label Lingo

Just about every packaged food made in the United States has a food label indicating serving size, nutritional information, and ingredients. Unfortunately, this critical piece of information is often overlooked, leading to unhealthy food choices that could have easily been avoided. In this chapter we will explore the elements of the food label as a guide to health.

Examining Ingredients

The very first thing you should do when deciding on a product is look at the ingredient list. This is the most detailed information on what a product contains and can help to answer the following questions.

❖ **Are the fats used in this product healthful or harmful?** Remember to look for foods made with olive, canola, or other healthful oils and avoid partially hydrogenated oils. This is of particular concern for packaged cereals, cookies, crackers, microwave popcorn, pastry, cake mixes, chips, and other cereal products but also applies to soups, frozen foods, and other premade convenience foods. Please refer to Chapter 4 to learn about your friends and foes of the fat world.

❖ **Is the product made with whole grains?** As we mentioned in Chapter 4, carbs help to balance blood sugar. If the label does not say "whole," the product is made with refined flour. Instead of "wheat flour," for example, look for "whole-wheat flour." This also applies for all other grains.

❖ **How much of each ingredient does the product contain?** The ingredient list is in descending order. The farther down the list you go, the less of that ingredient the product contains.

❖ **Is the product full of sugar?** Avoid products with high fructose corn syrup, as well as fruit sweeteners appearing high on the ingredient list. Although sugars from fruits in nature may be more healthful when consumed in their natural state (e.g., as part of that Red Delicious apple), juice concentrate sweeteners have the same effect on blood sugar and same number of calories as pure sugar.

❖ **How much of the product is actually a fruit or vegetable?** Although the product may be called "Strawberry Crunchies," after reading the food label you may find only a trace of strawberry flavor toward the end of the list. Choose foods that are nutrient dense and stay away from those that are merely empty calories.

Serving Size

Serving sizes are based on the amount of food people typically eat. However, many products contain multiple servings per package. Individual snack foods, for example, may contain 100 calories "per serving," but when you read the "Number of Servings" you find that energy bar you just ate contains three servings at 100 calories per serving, totaling 300 calories as opposed to the 100 you may have assumed. It doesn't just affect calories but also the amounts of all other nutritional components like fat, sugar, and salt.

Calories and Total Fat

Look at calories and focus on where those calories come from. Use your calories as you would a daily stipend and try to make the most of each. Are your calories coming from good-quality fats and whole grains, or are they derived from sugars or saturated and trans fats?

The total fat panel provides the total amount of fat per serving and also breaks down the amount and type of each. Although trans fats may not be listed here yet on many products, you can roughly estimate how much trans fat is in a product with a simple math equation.

By adding the saturated fat, monounsaturated fat, and polyunsaturated fats and subtracting them from the total fat, you will determine the grams of trans fat in a specific product. For example, look at Smart Balance Popcorn. The total fat is 9 grams. The saturated fat is 3.5 grams, the monounsaturated fat is 2.5 grams, and the polyunsaturated fat is 3 grams.

9 − (3.5 grams saturated + 2.5 grams monounsaturated
fat + 3 grams polyunsaturated fat) = 0 grams trans fat

Talk with your doctor regarding what percentage of calories
in your diet should come from fat, depending on your particular
nutrition needs.

Cholesterol and Daily Values

Cholesterol in your diest can raise your blood cholesterol level,
although usually not as much as saturated fat. Because dietary
cholesterol is found only in foods that come from animals, by
choosing plenty of fruits, vegetables, and whole grains, you can
stay under the daily 300 milligrams recommended by the American Heart Association.

Look at Label Claims

Another aspect of food labeling is label claims. Three types of
claims can be used for foods and dietary supplements: health
claims, nutrient content claims, and structure/function claims.

Health claims describe a relationship between a food, food
component, or dietary supplement ingredient and its effect on
reducing the risk of a particular disease or health-related condition.

Nutrient content claims characterize the level of nutrient in
a food product using terms such as *free*, *light*, and *low* or they compare the level of a nutrient in a food to that of another food, using
terms such as *more*, *reduced*, or *light*. These requirements ensure
that terms are used consistently for all products and are useful to
consumers. However, it's important to appreciate that sometimes
the so-called "good" and "excellent" sources of nutrients may not
be consistent or uniformly defined. This will give you a practical
tool to help make sound nutritional choices regarding diet.

Structure/function claims describe the role of a nutrient or dietary ingredient intended to affect normal structure or function in humans. Examples of structure/function claims include "calcium builds strong bones," "fiber maintains bowel regularity," and "antioxidants maintain cell integrity." You will find these types of claims on "functional foods" that may be fortified, such as fiber laxatives and some supplements.

FDA Approved Health Claims Relating to Diabetes. Here are some of the claims relevant to diabetes and heart disease. Please visit fda.gov for more information.

✽ **Dietary saturated fat and cholesterol and risk of coronary heart disease.** "While many factors affect heart disease, diets low in saturated fat and cholesterol may reduce the risk of this disease."

✽ **Fruits, vegetables, and grain products that contain fiber, particularly soluble fiber, and risk of coronary heart disease.** "Diets low in saturated fat and cholesterol and rich in fruits, vegetables, and grain products that contain some types of dietary fiber, particularly soluble fiber, may reduce the risk of heart disease, a disease associated with many factors."

✽ **Soy protein and risk of coronary heart disease.** "Diets low in saturated fat and cholesterol that include 25 grams of soy protein a day may reduce the risk of heart disease."

✽ **Plant sterol/stanol esters and risk of coronary heart disease.** "Diets low in saturated fat and cholesterol that include two servings of foods that provide a daily total of at least 3.4 grams of plant stanol esters in two meals may reduce the risk of heart disease."

✽ **Whole-grain foods and risk of heart disease and certain cancers.** "Diets rich in whole-grain foods and other plant foods and low in total fat, saturated fat, and cholesterol may reduce the risk of heart disease and some cancers."

Culinary Cautions

In the previous chapters, we have reviewed the research in support of fruits, vegetables, whole-grain products, and other plant foods for their role in diabetes prevention and management, as well as those foods, or food components, that may worsen diabetes or contribute to complications. This list summarizes many of the culinary cautions to take, based on the most current scientific research. Refer to individual Chapters 1, 4, and 5 for details.

* ❖ Red meats
* ❖ Processed or cured meats
* ❖ Alcohol
* ❖ Trans fats
* ❖ Saturated fats
* ❖ Sugars
* ❖ Refined grain products

Now that you're armed with powerful information on the healing nutrients of certain foods, it's time to put all of this information to use in the delicious and healthy meal plans and recipes courtesy of Healing Gourmet. Eat your medicine!

9

My Daily Dose: Meal Plans to Get You Started

You DON'T HAVE to be a master chef to be a Healing Gourmet. Just let the principles and recipes in this book guide you. We have included recipes suited for the culinary novice, for those pressed for time, and for those who want to maintain their healthy weight or lose weight—and we do it without sacrificing any flavor. Mealtime should be one of the most enjoyable of your day, so let us help you to make it healthy!

In this section, you will find seven-day meal plans for three different calorie levels—1,200, 1,600, and 2,000 calories. We recognize that readers will have different goals for their overall nutrition. These meal plans are only intended for use as a guide or template for meals and snacks. The right calorie level for an individual depends on his or her height, age, activity level, and goals for nutrition. For example, if you are carrying excess weight or are currently inactive, you may consider the 1,200- or 1,600-calorie menus. On the other hand, if you are active and have a healthy body weight, the 2,000-calorie menu may work for you. To help select an appropriate calorie level for you, we recommend you schedule an appointment with your registered dietitian or physician.

Each of these meal plans incorporates the science of good nutrition that you've just read into practical, flavorful, and easy recipes that you can put together for yourself or your family. However, no matter what your calorie level is, each of these levels incorporates the following healthy principles of diet planning:

* Use a variety of *lean protein sources* (averaging 20 to 25 percent of calories), limiting high fatty cuts of meat, incorporating fish, and encouraging "meatless" meals throughout the week.
* Emphasize *healthy fats*, using monounsaturated and polyunsaturated fats as your primary fat source—averaging 22 to 30 percent of total calories.
* Incorporate *healthy, whole-grain carbohydrates* (averaging 50 to 60 percent of total calories) for optimal blood sugar control.

The meal plans all limit or avoid the following:

* Saturated fats are minimized—averaging less than 7 percent of calories—trying at all times to eliminate trans fats from partially hydrogenated oils.
* Levels of dietary cholesterol are low to moderate (most days less than 200 mg/day).
* Sodium intake is moderate, with most days being less than 3,000 milligrams.

Finally, all these meal plans encourage you to:

* Consume a variety of foods—especially fruits, vegetables, and whole grains. (Remember, go for a variety of color and texture in your food choices.)
* Eat plenty of fruits and vegetables.

❖ Use whole grains as the main choice for breads, cereals, crackers, and pasta.

❖ Consume foods high in fiber—with a minimum of 25 grams per day.

❖ Use whole foods, free-range poultry, locally grown produce, and fresh herbs and spices.

Throughout this chapter, you'll find meals for breakfast, lunch, and dinner, as well as snacks to eat throughout the day. We include information about the nutritional content for the day, and use recipes from Chapter 10 (indicated with an asterisk*). You'll also find a Veg Out option for the non–meat eaters. While the nutrients (protein, fat, carbohydrate, and so forth) will be different than the ones used in the meal plans, the Veg Out option is a good vegetarian alternative. However, please check with your doctor or health-care provider before embarking on any of these meal plans to find out which one is right for you.

We also recommend drinking six to eight eight-ounce glasses of water a day. You can substitute low-sodium sparkling water for two of the six glasses a day and spring water with a lemon wedge to add some variety. Enjoy the variety of flavors, textures, and most of all the health benefits our foods have to offer!

My Meal Plans: 1,200 Calories

This low-calorie plan provides all the nutrients and phytonutrients you need while helping you to shed pounds. Discuss a calorie range that makes sense for your personal needs with your dietitian.

Day 1

BREAKFAST
½ cup old-fashioned oats (prepared according to directions with
   water) topped with
½ cup frozen unsweetened blueberries
Spring water

MIDMORNING SNACK
1 cup cinnamon apple tea
4 ounces nonfat light yogurt

LUNCH
2 ounces canned tuna in water, drained, combined with
3 cups fresh baby spinach
¼ cup sliced red onion
¼ cup sliced mushrooms
Four cherry tomatoes and
2 tablespoons light vinaigrette salad dressing
Spring water

MIDAFTERNOON SNACK
One medium apple with ½ teaspoon cinnamon
½ ounce dry-roasted peanuts

DINNER
One serving Pasta with Chicken and Veggies*
1 cup tossed greens topped with
1 tablespoon light vinaigrette dressing
1 cup decaffeinated green tea with lemon

Veg Out! *Try our Tempeh Cacciatore for a tempting veggie alternative.*

SNACK
½ cup nonfat sugar-free pudding
1 cup cinnamon apple tea

Nutrition information: 1,220 calories, 77 grams protein, 33 grams total fat, 6 grams saturated fat, 105 milligrams cholesterol, 165 grams carbohydrate, 20 grams dietary fiber, 1,300 milligrams sodium

Day 2

BREAKFAST
Two Kashi Go Lean frozen waffles topped with
One half medium banana, sliced, and
2 tablespoons sugar-free syrup
1 cup decaffeinated coffee

MIDMORNING SNACK
1 cup herbal tea
One medium orange

LUNCH
Homemade "pizza": in toaster oven, heat one small whole-wheat pita topped with 2 ounces marinara sauce, 2 ounces part-skim mozzarella cheese, and 1 cup sliced red, yellow, and green peppers
2 tablespoons light ranch dressing to dip

MIDAFTERNOON SNACK
¼ cup unsalted soy nuts

DINNER
One serving Salmon over Dandelion Greens with Garlic Soy
   Salsa*
½ cup cooked brown rice
1 cup green tea

Veg Out! *Try our Asian Tofu Cakes for a meatless alternative with Asian flavor.*

SNACK
6 ounces nonfat light fruit yogurt

Nutrition information: 1,220 calories, 69 grams protein, 41 grams total fat, 10 grams saturated fat, 100 milligrams cholesterol, 152 grams carbohydrate, 29 grams dietary fiber, 1,770 milligrams sodium

---

Day 3

BREAKFAST
1 cup Kashi Go Lean Cereal with
1 cup skim milk and
2 tablespoons raisins
1 cup decaffeinated coffee

MIDMORNING SNACK
One half grapefruit

LUNCH
One serving Mediterranean Spinach Pie*
One half small whole-wheat pita bread
Low-sodium sparkling water with lemon wedge

MIDAFTERNOON SNACK
½ cup 1 percent cottage cheese
½ ounce dry-roasted almonds

DINNER
4 ounces baked tilapia
1 cup steamed green beans
1 small sweet potato topped with
2 teaspoons trans fat–free tub margarine
Spring water

Veg Out! *Try our Bean and Veggie Soup with vegetable broth for ladles of protection and lots of fiber.*

SNACK
Two fat-free or trans fat–free Fig Newton cookies
1 cup cinnamon apple tea (herbal/decaffeinated)

Nutrition information: 1,180 calories, 88 grams protein, 26 grams total fat, 8 grams saturated fat, 230 milligrams cholesterol, 162 grams carbohydrate, 30 grams dietary fiber, 1,500 milligrams sodium

---

Day 4

BREAKFAST
One whole-wheat English muffin toasted under broiler or
　　toaster oven and topped with
½ cup 1 percent cottage cheese spread and
½ cup sliced strawberries and a dash of cinnamon
1 cup coffee with nonfat creamer

MIDMORNING SNACK
1 cup decaffeinated green tea with ½ teaspoon cinnamon or cinnamon apple tea (herbal/decaffeinated)

LUNCH
One large ripe tomato cored and stuffed with
¼ cup leftover brown rice
2 ounces diced chicken
2 tablespoons light mayonnaise and
1 cup mixed diced celery and onion
Spring water

MIDAFTERNOON SNACK
1 cup cinnamon apple tea (herbal/decaffeinated)

DINNER
One serving Stuffed Eggplant with Peanut Sauce*
One slice whole-grain crusty bread topped with
2 teaspoons light trans fat–free margarine
1 cup herbal tea

SNACK
1 cup berries topped with
2 tablespoons nonfat whipped topping
Decaffeinated green tea with lemon

Nutrition information: 1,220 calories, 62 grams protein, 24 grams total fat, 3 grams saturated fat, 65 grams cholesterol, 201 grams carbohydrate, 36 grams dietary fiber, 2,120 milligrams sodium

Day 5

BREAKFAST
One Apple and Date Muffin* topped with
2 teaspoons natural peanut butter
1 cup skim milk

MIDMORNING SNACK
One medium pear
1 cup herbal tea

LUNCH
3 cups tossed salad greens topped with
¼ cup shredded carrots
¼ cup sliced cucumbers
¼ cup diced celery
2 ounces baked barbeque-flavored tofu and
2 tablespoons light salad dressing
Spring water

MIDAFTERNOON SNACK
1 cup cut-up fresh vegetables

DINNER
6 ounces roast turkey
One small baked potato with skin topped with
¼ cup fresh salsa
2 cups steamed spinach and red peppers
1 cup iced decaffeinated green tea

Veg Out! *Try our Crunchy Lentil Salad for a healthy dose of blood-sugar balancing phytoestrogens and fiber.*

Snack
Cinnamon apple tea (herbal/decaffeinated)

Nutrition information: 1,230 calories, 62 grams protein, 45 grams total fat, 10 grams saturated fat, 115 milligrams cholesterol, 156 grams carbohydrates, 26 grams dietary fiber, 1,370 milligrams sodium

---

Day 6

Breakfast
4 egg white omelet filled with
1 cup raw spinach, sautéed in cooking spray and
2 tablespoons rehydrated sun-dried tomatoes
One slice whole-wheat toast topped with
1 teaspoon trans fat–free tub margarine
1 cup green tea

Midmorning Snack
One tangerine

Lunch
1 cup Bean and Veggie Soup*
One slice cracked-wheat bread filled with
2 ounces lemon pepper turkey breast, lettuce, tomato, and
2 teaspoons Dijon mustard
One medium apple with ½ teaspoon cinnamon
1 cup herbal tea

Midafternoon Snack
One granola bar (2 grams or more fiber, less than 15 grams
    sugar)
4 ounces skim milk

DINNER
One serving Risotto Tart with Tomatoes, Onions, and Peppers*
1½ cups tossed mixed greens mixed with
¼ cup sliced radish
¼ cup sliced carrot
¼ cup diced celery and
2 tablespoons balsamic vinaigrette dressing
Spring water

SNACK
Herbal tea

Nutrition information: 1,260 calories, 71 grams protein, 35 grams total fat, 6 grams saturated fat, 45 milligrams cholesterol, 177 grams carbohydrate, 28 grams dietary fiber, 3,310 milligrams sodium

Day 7

BREAKFAST
One slice Vegetable Frittata*
6 ounces low-sodium vegetable juice

MIDMORNING SNACK
6 ounces light fruit yogurt

LUNCH
1 cup vegetarian chili topped with
2 tablespoons 2 percent fat, reduced sodium shredded cheddar
   cheese
Five whole-grain crackers

MIDAFTERNOON SNACK
Ten dry-roasted almonds
One medium pear

DINNER
One serving Spicy Turkey Meatloaf with Spinach*
½ cup garlic mashed potatoes
1½ cups steamed asparagus
Spring water

Veg Out! *Try our Mediterranean Spinach Pie for a slice of health.*

SNACK
½ cup low-fat vanilla yogurt

Nutrition information: 1,250 calories, 79 grams protein, 32 grams total fat, 9 grams saturated fat, 240 milligrams cholesterol, 177 grams carbohydrate, 41 grams dietary fiber, 2,440 milligrams sodium

---

My Meal Plans: 1,600 Calories

This plan still offers a calorie range that will help some people lose weight, depending, of course, on the factors we discussed previously. Your doctor can tell you if this plan may be right for you.

Day 1

BREAKFAST
½ cup old-fashioned oats (prepared according to directions with water) topped with
1 cup frozen unsweetened blueberries
¼ cup nonfat plain yogurt topped with

2 tablespoons ground walnuts
1 cup herbal tea

MIDMORNING SNACK
1 cup decaffeinated black tea with ½ teaspoon cinnamon or cinnamon apple tea (herbal/decaffeinated)
6 ounces nonfat cottage cheese

LUNCH
3 ounces canned tuna in water, drained, combined with
3 cups fresh baby spinach
¼ cup sliced red onion
¼ cup sliced mushrooms
Four cherry tomatoes and
2 tablespoons light vinaigrette salad dressing
One sprouted-grain roll
Spring water

MIDAFTERNOON SNACK
One medium apple with ½ teaspoon cinnamon
1½ ounces 2 percent cheddar cheese

DINNER
One serving Pasta with Chicken and Veggies*
2 cups tossed greens topped with
2 tablespoons light vinaigrette dressing
Spring water

Veg Out! *Try our Pasta with Asparagus and Lemon for a similar meal, minus the meat.*

SNACK
½ cup nonfat sugar-free pudding
Cinnamon apple tea (herbal/decaffeinated)

Nutrition information: 1,580 calories, 105 grams protein, 43 grams total fat, 9 grams saturated fat, 125 milligrams cholesterol, 208 grams carbohydrate, 24 grams dietary fiber, 2,040 milligrams sodium

Day 2

BREAKFAST
Two Kashi Go Lean frozen waffles topped with
One medium banana, sliced, and
2 tablespoons sugar-free syrup
One 2-ounce vegetarian sausage patty
1 cup decaffeinated coffee with nonfat creamer

MIDMORNING SNACK
One medium orange
1 cup herbal tea

LUNCH
Homemade "pizza": in toaster oven, heat one small whole-wheat
    pita topped with 2 ounces marinara sauce, 3 ounces sliced
    chicken, 2 ounces part-skim mozzarella cheese, and 1 cup
    sliced red, yellow, and green peppers
2 tablespoons light ranch dressing to dip
Spring water

MIDAFTERNOON SNACK
6 ounces nonfat light fruit yogurt

DINNER
One serving Salmon over Dandelion Greens with Garlic Soy
    Salsa*
½ cup cooked brown rice

1 cup steamed broccoli topped with
1 tablespoon grated parmesan cheese
1 cup decaffeinated green tea

Veg Out! *Try our Risotto Tart with Tomatoes, Onions, and Peppers and some minestrone soup for a meatless meal with Mediterranean appeal.*

SNACK
¼ cup unsalted soy nuts
1 cup cinnamon apple tea (herbal/decaffeinated)

Nutrition information: 1,590 calories, 115 grams protein, 48 grams total fat, 13 grams saturated fat, 180 milligrams cholesterol, 187 grams carbohydrate, 37 grams dietary fiber, 2,390 milligrams sodium

Day 3

BREAKFAST
1 cup Kashi Go Lean cereal with
1 cup skim milk and
2 tablespoons raisins
One slice whole-grain toast topped with
2 teaspoons natural peanut butter
1 cup decaffeinated coffee with nonfat creamer

MIDMORNING SNACK
One grapefruit

LUNCH
One serving Mediterranean Spinach Pie*
One half small whole-wheat pita
Low-sodium sparkling water with lemon wedge

MIDAFTERNOON SNACK
½ cup 1 percent cottage cheese
½ ounce dry-roasted almonds

DINNER
4 ounces baked tilapia
2 cups steamed green beans
One small sweet potato topped with
2 teaspoons trans fat–free tub margarine
Spring water

Veg Out! *Try our Vegetable Lettuce Rolls for a colorful array of veggies.*

SNACK
Five gingersnap cookies
8 ounces chocolate soy milk

Nutrition information: 1,600 calories, 104 grams protein, 44 grams total fat, 11 grams saturated fat, 230 milligrams cholesterol, 220 grams carbohydrate, 47 grams dietary fiber, 1,690 milligrams sodium

---

Day 4

BREAKFAST
One whole-wheat English muffin toasted under broiler or
    toaster oven and topped with
½ cup 1 percent cottage cheese spread and
¾ cup sliced strawberries and ¼ teaspoon cinnamon
1 cup coffee with nonfat creamer

MIDMORNING SNACK
Two whole-wheat graham crackers topped with
2 teaspoons almond butter

LUNCH
One large ripe tomato cored and stuffed with
¼ cup leftover brown rice
3 ounces diced chicken
2 tablespoons light mayonnaise and
1 cup mixed diced celery and onion
Five whole-grain crackers

MIDAFTERNOON SNACK
One part-skim mozzarella string cheese stick
Decaffeinated green tea with lemon

DINNER
One serving Stuffed Eggplant with Peanut Sauce*
One slice whole-grain crusty bread topped with
2 teaspoons light trans fat–free margarine
1 cup berries topped with
2 tablespoons nonfat whipped topping
Spring water

SNACK
One medium apple with ½ teaspoon cinnamon

Nutrition information: 1,630 calories, 83 grams protein, 41 grams total fat, 8 grams saturated fat, 105 grams cholesterol, 249 grams carbohydrate, 43 grams dietary fiber, 2,650 milligrams sodium

Day 5

BREAKFAST
One Apple and Date Muffin* topped with
2 teaspoons natural peanut butter
1 cup skim milk
1 cup coffee

MIDMORNING SNACK
One medium pear
½ cup 1 percent cottage cheese
1 cup herbal tea

LUNCH
3 cups tossed salad greens topped with
¼ cup shredded carrots
¼ cup sliced cucumbers
¼ cup diced celery
3 ounces baked barbeque-flavored tofu and
2 tablespoons light salad dressing
1 ounce whole wheat pretzels
Spring water

MIDAFTERNOON SNACK
1 cup cut-up fresh vegetables
¼ cup red pepper hummus
Herbal tea

DINNER
6 ounces roast turkey
One small baked potato with skin topped with
¼ cup fresh salsa
2 cups steamed spinach and red peppers
Spring water

Veg Out! *Try our Mediterranean Spinach Pie for a slice of health.*

SNACK
½ cup 1 percent cottage cheese
Decaffeinated black tea with ½ teaspoon cinnamon

Nutrition information: 1,570 calories, 88 grams protein, 55 grams total fat, 12 grams saturated fat, 120 milligrams cholesterol, 193 grams carbohydrate, 33 grams dietary fiber, 1,230 milligrams sodium

---

Day 6

BREAKFAST
4 egg white omelet filled with
1 cup raw spinach, sautéed in cooking spray and
2 tablespoons rehydrated sun-dried tomatoes
Two slices whole-wheat toast topped with
2 teaspoons trans fat–free tub margarine
One tangerine
Green tea

MIDMORNING SNACK
1 ounce unsalted dry-roasted peanuts

LUNCH
1 cup Bean and Veggie Soup*
One slice cracked-wheat bread filled with
3 ounces lemon pepper turkey breast, lettuce, tomato, and
2 teaspoons Dijon mustard
One medium apple with ½ teaspoon cinnamon

MIDAFTERNOON SNACK
One granola bar (2 grams or more fiber, less than 15 grams
   sugar)
4 ounces skim milk

DINNER
One serving Risotto Tart with Tomatoes, Onions, and Peppers*
1½ cups tossed mixed greens mixed with
¼ cup sliced radish
¼ cup sliced carrot
¼ cup diced celery
2 tablespoons balsamic vinaigrette dressing
Spring water

SNACK
1 cup no-sugar-added hot chocolate

Nutrition information: 1,570 calories, 84 grams protein, 51 grams total
fat, 8 grams saturated fat, 45 milligrams cholesterol, 209 grams
carbohydrate, 33 grams dietary fiber, 3,690 milligrams sodium

---

Day 7

BREAKFAST
One slice Vegetable Frittata*
6 ounces low-sodium vegetable juice
1 cup cubed melon
Herbal tea

MIDMORNING SNACK
6 ounces light fruit yogurt

LUNCH
1 cup vegetarian chili topped with
2 tablespoons 2 percent reduced-sodium shredded cheddar
  cheese
Five whole-grain crackers
1 cup herbal tea

MIDAFTERNOON SNACK
Ten dry-roasted almonds
One medium pear

DINNER
One serving Spicy Turkey Meatloaf with Spinach*
1 cup garlic mashed potatoes
1½ cups steamed asparagus topped with
1 teaspoon olive oil
Spring water

Veg Out! *Try our Vegetarian Paella as a one-pot meal that delivers a spectrum of phytonutrients and six and a half servings of veggies!*

SNACK
½ cup low-fat vanilla yogurt topped with
2 teaspoons crushed walnuts and
2 tablespoons nonfat whipped topping
Herbal tea

Nutrition information: 1,600 calories, 85 grams protein, 52 grams total fat, 14 grams saturated fat, 255 milligrams cholesterol, 214 grams carbohydrate, 44 grams dietary fiber, 2,860 milligrams sodium

---

My Meal Plans: 2,000 Calories

This plan is typically suitable for those seeking to maintain their weight. Again, we emphasize, please consult your physician.

Day 1

BREAKFAST

¾ cup old-fashioned oats (prepared according to directions with
  water) topped with
1 cup fresh or frozen unsweetened blueberries
¼ cup nonfat plain yogurt topped with
2 tablespoons ground walnuts
1 cup black tea with ½ teaspoon cinnamon

MIDMORNING SNACK

6 ounces nonfat cottage cheese
¼ cup whole-grain crunchy cereal

LUNCH

3 ounces canned tuna in water, drained, combined with
3 cups fresh baby spinach
¼ cup sliced red onion
¼ cup sliced mushrooms
Four cherry tomatoes
2 tablespoons part-skim mozzarella cheese and
2 tablespoons light vinaigrette dressing
One sprouted-grain roll
Spring water

MIDAFTERNOON SNACK

One medium apple with ½ teaspoon cinnamon
1½ ounces 2 percent cheddar cheese

DINNER

One and a half servings Pasta with Chicken and Veggies*
2 cups tossed greens topped with
2 tablespoons light vinaigrette dressing
1 cup herbal tea

Veg Out! *Try our Penne with Portobello and Veggie Sausage for a bite that's full of phyte!*

SNACK

½ cup nonfat sugar-free pudding
1 cup cinnamon apple tea

Nutrition information: 2,080 calories, 138 grams protein, 57 grams total fat, 15 grams saturated fat, 180 milligrams cholesterol, 271 grams carbohydrate, 31 grams dietary fiber, 2,590 milligrams sodium

---

Day 2

BREAKFAST

2 Kashi Go Lean frozen waffles topped with
One medium banana, sliced
2 tablespoons sugar-free syrup and
2 teaspoons light trans fat–free margarine
One 2-ounce vegetarian sausage patty
1 cup decaffeinated coffee

MIDMORNING SNACK

1 cup herbal tea with ½ teaspoon cinnamon
¼ cup trail mix
One medium orange

LUNCH

Homemade "pizza": in toaster oven, heat one small whole-wheat
   pita topped with 2 ounces marinara sauce, 3 ounces sliced
   chicken, 2 ounces part-skim mozzarella cheese, and 1 cup
   sliced red, yellow, and green peppers
2 tablespoons light ranch dressing to dip
1 cup skim milk

MIDAFTERNOON SNACK

6 ounces nonfat light fruit yogurt
1 cup cinnamon apple tea (herbal/decaffeinated)

DINNER

One serving Salmon over Dandelion Greens with Garlic Soy
   Salsa*
1 cup cooked brown rice
1 cup steamed broccoli topped with
1 tablespoon grated parmesan cheese
1 cup mixed berries
1 cup herbal tea

Veg Out! *Try our Tempeh Cacciatore for a tempting veggie alternative.*

SNACK

¼ cup unsalted soy nuts
Decaffeinated green tea with ½ teaspoon cinnamon

Nutrition information: 1,960 calories, 129 grams protein, 63 grams
total fat, 15 grams saturated fat, 185 milligrams cholesterol, 237 grams
carbohydrate, 42 grams dietary fiber, 2,560 milligrams sodium

---

Day 3

BREAKFAST
1 cup Kashi Go Lean cereal with
1 cup skim milk and
2 tablespoons raisins
One half medium banana
One slice whole-grain toast topped with
1 tablespoon natural peanut butter
1 cup decaffeinated coffee

MIDMORNING SNACK
One grapefruit

LUNCH
One and a half servings Mediterranean Spinach Pie*
One small whole-wheat pita
Low-sodium sparkling water with lemon wedge

MIDAFTERNOON SNACK
1 ounce dry-roasted almonds
6 ounces light fruit yogurt

DINNER
6 ounces baked tilapia
2 cups steamed green beans
One small sweet potato topped with
2 teaspoons trans fat–free tub margarine
1 cup herbal tea

Veg Out! *Try our Asian Tofu Cakes for a meatless alternative with Asian flavor.*

SNACK
Five gingersnap cookies
8 ounces chocolate soy milk

Nutrition information: 1,980 calories, 123 grams protein, 60 grams total fat, 14 grams saturated fat, 340 milligrams cholesterol, 265 grams carbohydrate, 53 grams dietary fiber, 1,700 milligrams sodium

---

Day 4

BREAKFAST
One whole-wheat English muffin toasted under broiler or
  toaster oven and topped with
½ cup 1 percent cottage cheese spread and
¾ cup sliced strawberries and ¼ teaspoon cinnamon
1 cup decaffeinated coffee with nonfat creamer

MIDMORNING SNACK
One part-skim mozzarella string cheese stick
Herbal tea

LUNCH
One large red ripe tomato cored and stuffed with
½ cup brown rice mixed with
3 ounces canned salmon or chicken
2 tablespoons light mayonnaise and
4 tablespoons diced celery and onion
Seven reduced-fat woven-wheat crackers
Spring water

MIDAFTERNOON SNACK
1 ounce walnuts
1 cup green or black tea

DINNER
One serving Stuffed Eggplant with Peanut Sauce*
One slice whole-grain crusty bread topped with
2 teaspoons light trans fat–free margarine
2 cups sliced red onion, tomato, and cucumber topped with
2 tablespoons feta cheese,
2 teaspoons olive oil, and
1 tablespoon balsamic vinegar
1 cup fresh fruit salad (blueberries, strawberries, melon) topped
   with
2 tablespoons nonfat, nonhydrogenated whipped topping
1 cup herbal tea

SNACK
One medium apple with ½ teaspoon cinnamon

Nutrition information: 2,010 calories, 100 grams protein, 67 grams total fat, 15 grams saturated fat, 80 grams cholesterol, 272 grams carbohydrate, 48 grams dietary fiber, 3,470 milligrams sodium

---

Day 5

BREAKFAST
Two Apple and Date Muffins* topped with
1 tablespoon natural peanut butter
1 cup skim milk
1 cup coffee

MIDMORNING SNACK
One medium pear
½ cup 1 percent cottage cheese
Herbal tea

LUNCH
3 cups tossed salad greens topped with
¼ cup shredded carrots
¼ cup sliced cucumbers
¼ cup diced celery
4 ounces baked barbeque flavored tofu and
2 tablespoons light salad dressing
1 ounce whole-wheat pretzels
Spring water

MIDAFTERNOON SNACK
1 cup cut up fresh vegetables
¼ cup red pepper hummus
1 cup herbal tea

DINNER
6 ounces roast turkey
One small baked potato with skin topped with
¼ cup fresh salsa
2 cups steamed spinach and red peppers
Spring water

Veg Out! *Try our Pasta with Asparagus and Lemon for a similar meal, minus the meat.*

SNACK
3 cups popped light microwave popcorn (trans fat free)
Cinnamon apple tea (herbal/decaffeinated)

Nutrition information: 2,080 calories, 104 grams protein, 78 grams total fat, 15 grams saturated fat, 155 milligrams cholesterol, 254 grams carbohydrate, 44 grams dietary fiber, 2,790 milligrams sodium

Day 6

BREAKFAST
4 egg white omelet filled with
1 cup raw spinach sautéed in cooking spray
2 tablespoons sun-dried tomatoes and
1 ounce reduced-fat feta cheese
Two slices whole-wheat toast topped with
2 teaspoons trans fat–free tub margarine
One tangerine
Green tea

MIDMORNING SNACK
1 ounce unsalted dry-roasted peanuts
2 tablespoons dried cranberries

LUNCH
1 cup Bean and Veggie Soup*
1 whole-wheat tortilla rolled with
3 ounces reduced-sodium turkey breast, lettuce, tomato, and
2 teaspoons Dijon mustard
One medium apple with ½ teaspoon cinnamon
1 cup herbal tea

MIDAFTERNOON SNACK
One granola bar (2 grams or more fiber, fewer than 15 grams
    sugar)
8 ounces skim milk

DINNER
One and a half servings Risotto Tart with Tomatoes, Onions,
    and Peppers*
1½ cups tossed mixed greens mixed with

¼ cup sliced radish
¼ cup sliced carrot
¼ cup diced celery
2 teaspoons olive oil and
2 tablespoons rice wine vinegar
Spring water

SNACK
1 ounce dark chocolate

Nutrition information: 2,020 calories, 103 grams protein, 67 grams total fat, 17 grams saturated fat, 60 milligrams cholesterol, 279 grams carbohydrate, 39 grams dietary fiber, 3,610 milligrams sodium

---

Day 7

BREAKFAST
One slice Vegetable Frittata*
6 ounces low-sodium vegetable juice
1 cup cubed melon
1 slice hearty rye bread
1 cup herbal tea

MIDMORNING SNACK
6 ounces light fruit yogurt

LUNCH
2 cups vegetarian chili topped with
2 tablespoons 2 percent, reduced-sodium shredded cheddar
    cheese
Five whole-grain crackers

1 cup sliced mango
1 cup herbal tea

MIDAFTERNOON SNACK
Ten dry-roasted almonds
One medium pear

DINNER
One serving Spicy Turkey Meatloaf with Spinach*
1 cup garlic mashed potatoes
1½ cups steamed asparagus topped with
1 teaspoon olive oil

Veg Out! *Keep your diabetes under wraps with our Vegetable Lettuce Rolls*

SNACK
½ cup low-fat vanilla yogurt topped with
2 teaspoons crushed walnuts and
2 tablespoons nonfat whipped topping
Herbal tea

Nutrition information: 2,010 calories, 110 grams protein, 59 grams total fat, 18 grams saturated fat, 270 milligrams cholesterol, 280 grams carbohydrate, 60 grams dietary fiber, 3,700 sodium

10

Gourmet Rx:
The Recipes

Now that you've learned about all of the wonderfully delicious foods that can help stabilize your blood sugar and prevent many of the complications associated with diabetes, let's put it into practice! Here you will find fifty recipes, suited for the novice chef, to cook your way to better health. In addition, we indicate when a meal is **Full of Fiber** ✢ which means that those particular recipes contain at least 5 grams of blood-sugar balancing fiber. Please note that the nutritional information does not include optional ingredients.

Soups and Salads

No longer revered as side items, soups and salads take a starring role in your health. Fresh vegetables and a variety of beans help protect your cells from oxidative damage.

❖ *Cream of Asparagus Soup (Full of Fiber)*

This soup is great served chilled on a warm spring day. The sea kelp or nori (toasted seaweed) can be found near the sushi area in your supermarket.

1 bunch of asparagus, cut into 2-inch pieces
1½ avocados
½ small onion, chopped
2 teaspoons tomatillo powder
3 celery stalks, strings peeled and chopped
6 sprigs organic parsley
Kelp or nori to taste
1 tablespoon fresh lime juice
½ cup fat-free plain yogurt
1 teaspoon sea salt

Bring two cups of water to a boil. Add the asparagus. Cook for 5 minutes. Strain and refresh under cold water. Asparagus should be bright green. Combine all the ingredients and 1 cup of water in a blender and process until creamy. Serve cold.

Serves 4 (serving size: 1 cup)

Servings of fruits and vegetables: 1.5 vegetables, 0.5 fruit; **diabetes-beating phytonutrients:** glutathione, quercetin, anthocyanins, saponins

Nutrition information: 160 calories, 6 grams protein, 10 grams total fat, 1.5 grams saturated fat, less than 1 milligram cholesterol, 16 grams carbohydrate, 8 grams dietary fiber, 641 milligrams sodium

✤ *Lemon Garbanzo Soup (Full of Fiber)*

Also known as "avgolemono," this soup marries blood-sugar balancing chickpeas and turmeric with veggies in a chicken broth for a light but hearty meal.

4 cups chicken or vegetable broth
1 16-ounce can chickpeas, drained
5 garlic cloves, chopped
⅛ teaspoon cumin seeds
½ teaspoon turmeric
2 egg whites
⅓ cup fresh lemon juice
1 teaspoon lemon zest
3 cups baby spinach
Pinch of cayenne pepper
Lemon slices for garnish

Combine broth, chickpeas, garlic, cumin, and turmeric in a large pot. Bring to a boil, reduce heat, and simmer for 15 minutes. Whisk eggs, lemon juice, and zest in bowl. Whisk 2 cups of hot soup into the egg white mixture. Add back to pot along with baby spinach, stirring over medium-low heat for 5 minutes. Add cayenne, ladle into bowls, float lemon slices atop, and serve.

Serves 4 (serving size: 1 cup)

Servings of fruits and vegetables: less than 0.5 vegetable; **diabetes-beating phytonutrients:** quercetin, beta-sitosterol, phytoestrogens, allicin, saponins, lignins, curcumin

Nutrition information: 150 calories, 12 grams protein, 1 gram total fat, no saturated fat, no cholesterol, 23 grams carbohydrate, 5 grams dietary fiber, 612 milligrams sodium

✣ *Tahinos Pumpkin Chowder (Full of Fiber)*

A carotenoid-rich soup that can be enjoyed either hot or cold. Make sure to keep the avocado cream chilled.

2 tablespoons olive oil
1 large red onion, chopped (about 1½ cups)
4 celery stalks, diced
1 1½-pound pumpkin or butternut squash, peeled and diced
3 cups canned chicken or vegetable broth
Sea salt
Freshly ground black pepper
1 large avocado, peeled and pitted
1 tablespoon fresh lime or lemon juice
1 bunch fresh cilantro, stems trimmed

Heat olive oil in a heavy, large saucepan over medium heat. Add chopped red onion and half of diced celery. Sauté until vegetables are tender, about 10 minutes. Add pumpkin or butternut squash and 2½ cups chicken or vegetable broth. Simmer until pumpkin is very tender, about 25 minutes. Working in batches, transfer soup to a food processor and puree until smooth. Season to taste with salt and pepper. Cover and refrigerate until well chilled.

Bring a small saucepan of salted water to boil. Add the remaining celery and cook for 2 minutes. Drain and chill. Mash avocado and lime or lemon juice in small bowl. Place fresh cilantro in blender with remaining ½ cup chicken broth. Blend until smooth. Mix 6 tablespoons cilantro puree into avocado mixture. Season to taste with sea salt and pepper. Ladle soup into bowls. Place small scoop of avocado mixture in center of each. Sprinkle soup with celery and serve.

Serves 4 (serving size: 1 cup)

Servings of fruits and vegetables: 2 vegetables; **diabetes-beating phytonutrients:** beta-carotene, quercetin, allylic sulfides, beta-sitosterol, anthocyanins, glutathione

Nutrition information: 270 calories, 5 grams protein, 15 grams total fat, 2 grams saturated fat, no cholesterol, 35 grams carbohydrate, 11 grams dietary fiber, 413 milligrams sodium

---

✢ *Bean and Veggie Soup (Full of Fiber)*

Ladles of protection! Blood-sugar balancing beans are the star of the show in this delicious soup.

1 tablespoon grapeseed oil
1 cup diced yellow onion
1 cup finely chopped red bell pepper
2 cloves garlic, crushed
4 cups chicken or vegetable broth

2 bay leaves
2 tablespoons chopped parsley
½ teaspoon freshly ground black pepper
1 teaspoon dry thyme
2 cups broccoli florets
1½ cups sliced carrots
1 15-ounce can garbanzo beans (chickpeas), drained

In a soup pot, heat oil over medium heat. Add onion and cook until translucent. Add red bell pepper, garlic, broth, bay leaves, parsley, black pepper, and thyme. Stir well. Add broccoli, carrots, and garbanzo beans. Simmer over medium heat for 20 minutes, so that vegetables are crisp tender and beans are firm.

Serves 4 (serving size: 1 cup)

Servings of fruits and vegetables: 3 vegetables; **diabetes-beating phytonutrients:** phytoestrogens, quercetin, beta-sitosterol, lignans, anthocyanins, kaempferol

Nutrition information: 217 calories, 9 grams protein, 6 grams total fat, no saturated fat, no cholesterol, 35 grams carbohydrate, 9 grams dietary fiber, 628 milligrams sodium

✦ *Crunchy Lentil Salad (Full of Fiber)*

Full of herbs, this lentil salad will make you love your legumes!

1 cup dried green or brown lentils, sorted and rinsed
2½ cups reduced-sodium, low-fat chicken or vegetable
broth

2 cups corn kernels

1 cup chopped celery

1 cup chopped flat-leaf parsley

¾ cup chopped red onion

¼ cup balsamic vinegar

3 tablespoons extra-virgin olive oil

1 tablespoon chopped fresh marjoram

3 teaspoons dried grated orange zest

1 teaspoon sea salt

¼ teaspoon freshly ground black pepper

Place lentils and broth in a medium saucepan. Bring to a boil then reduce heat to a simmer; cover and cook for 25 to 30 minutes or until tender. Lentils should absorb all the broth; if not, drain in colander. Transfer lentils to large bowl. Mix in corn, celery, parsley, and onion. Let cool. In a small bowl, whisk together vinegar, oil, marjoram, and orange zest. When lentil mixture is at room temperature, drizzle dressing over top and toss lightly to mix in. Add salt and pepper to taste, if desired. Serve cold or at room temperature.

Serves 4 (serving size: 2 cups)

Servings of fruits and vegetables: 1 vegetable; **diabetes-beating phytonutrients:** phytoestrogens, quercetin, beta-sitosterol, kaempferol, anthocyanins

Nutrition information: 400 calories, 19 grams protein, 11 grams total fat, 1.5 saturated fat, no cholesterol, 62 grams carbohydrate, 10 grams dietary fiber, 900 milligrams sodium (Note: If this amount of sodium is too high for your diet, you can omit the sea salt and cut it down to 320 milligrams!)

Dilled Chicken Salad Wrap

Health under wraps! This healthy sandwich provides whole grains and veggies along with vitamin B–rich chicken.

1 pound skinless, boneless chicken breasts
1½ cups chicken broth
3 tablespoons low-fat or fat-free yogurt
2 tablespoons grapeseed oil
2½ tablespoons chopped fresh dill
1 cup fresh asparagus spears
1 cup fresh spinach
½ teaspoon sea salt
½ teaspoon ground black pepper
4 8-inch whole-wheat flour tortillas

Poach chicken breasts in chicken broth for 20 minutes or until center is white. Remove from heat; drain and cool. Shred chicken and combine with yogurt, 1 tablespoon oil, and dill. In a separate pan, sauté asparagus and spinach in remaining 1 tablespoon oil for 2 minutes; asparagus should be crisp-tender and spinach should be bright green. Combine with chicken and mix well. Season with salt and pepper. Layer chicken mixture over tortilla; roll forming a wrap, cut in half diagonally, and serve.

Serves 4 (serving size: 1 wrap)

Servings of fruits and vegetables: 1 vegetable; **diabetes-beating phytonutrients:** glutathione, saponins, flavonoids, beta-carotene

Nutrition information: 287 calories, 32 grams protein, 9 grams total fat, 1 gram saturated fat, 66 milligrams cholesterol, 24 grams carbohydrate, 3.5 grams dietary fiber, 465 milligrams sodium

Tuna Salad with Broccoli, Red Peppers, and Vidalia Onion

An old standby gets a nutritional boost and a snappy crunch with peppers, onions, watercress, and broccoli. If watercress is not available, you can substitute arugula or baby salad mix.

2 cups flat-leafed spinach
1 cup watercress
2 cups broccoli florets
1 cup sliced red pepper
Canola oil spray
½ cup sliced Vidalia onion
2 6-ounce cans albacore tuna in water, drained well
3 tablespoons flaxseed or canola oil
3 tablespoons balsamic vinegar (optional)
Juice of 1 lemon
2 cloves garlic, crushed
Handful fresh basil, chopped
Freshly ground black pepper

Rinse spinach and watercress and layer in a salad bowl. Sauté broccoli and red peppers for 2 minutes in a sauté pan sprayed with oil. Remove from heat and set aside. Layer onions, broccoli, and red pepper over greens. Top with flaky albacore tuna. Mix oil, vinegar (if using), lemon juice, and garlic in a small bowl. Drizzle over salad; top with fresh basil and pepper.

Serves 2 as a light entrée (serving size: ½ recipe) or 4 as a salad course (serving size: ¼ recipe)

Servings of fruits and vegetables: 1 vegetable; **diabetes-beating phytonutrients:** phytoestrogens, quercetin, beta-carotene, anthocyanins

Nutrition information: 230 calories, 23 grams protein, 11 grams total fat, 1 gram saturated fat, 25 milligrams cholesterol, 11 grams carbohydrates, 2 grams dietary fiber, 310 milligrams sodium

Papaya, Red Onion, and Watercress Salad with Lemon Mint Dressing

Members of the allium and crucifer family team up with tropical papaya to deliver a healthy dose of antioxidants and phytonutrients. This salad can also work well with arugula if watercress is not available.

1 cup sliced papaya
¼ cup sliced red onion
2 cups spinach leaves
1 cup watercress
⅓ cup finely chopped fresh mint leaves
3 tablespoons fresh lemon juice
1 teaspoon lemon zest
¼ teaspoon cayenne pepper
2 tablespoons flaxseed oil

Arrange papaya and red onion over spinach and watercress. Mix mint with lemon juice, zest, cayenne peppers, and flaxseed oil.

Serves 4 (serving size: ¼ recipe)

Servings of fruits and vegetables: 0.5 vegetable, 0.5 fruit; **diabetes-beating phytonutrients:** quercetin, phytoestrogens, beta-carotene, saponins

Nutrition information: 88 calories, 1 gram protein, 7 grams total fat, 5 grams saturated fat, no cholesterol, 7 grams carbohydrates, 1.5 grams dietary fiber, 25 milligrams sodium

❖ *Spinach Salad with Figs, Red Onion, and Goat Cheese (Full of Fiber)*

You can substitute dry figs if fresh ones are not available.

6 cups flat-leafed baby spinach
1 cup sliced red onion
12 fresh figs, stems removed and halved
¼ cup goat cheese crumbles (or veggie cheese)
2 tablespoons extra-virgin olive oil
6 tablespoons balsamic vinegar

Add spinach to a salad bowl. Top with red onion, figs, and goat cheese crumbles. Mix oil and vinegar, drizzle over salad, and serve.

Serves 4 (serving size: ¼ recipe)

Servings of fruits and vegetables: 1.5 vegetables, 2.0 fruits; **diabetes-beating phytonutrients:** quercetin, beta-carotene, saponins, kaempferol

Nutrition information: 465 calories, 8.5 grams protein, 30 grams total fat, 9 grams saturated fat, 22 milligrams cholesterol, 45 grams carbohydrate, 6.5 grams dietary fiber, 211 milligrams sodium

Spicy Noodles Salad with Baked Tofu

Oh soy! This humble bean has a big role in preventing heart disease and helping to stabilize blood sugar. The baked tofu for this salad is available at the organic section in the produce department of your supermarket.

6 ounces dry rice noodles
9 ounces low-sodium baked tofu, cut into cubes
1 cup peeled, seeded, and thinly sliced cucumber
1 cup julienned red bell pepper
1 cup grated carrots
⅓ cup chopped scallions
½ cup chopped fresh cilantro
2 tablespoons chopped fresh basil
1 tablespoon chopped fresh mint
¼ cup rice wine vinegar
6 tablespoons reduced-sodium soy sauce
1 teaspoon dried red chili flakes
5 tablespoons sesame oil

Bring 3 cups of water to a boil. Pour over the rice noodles and let sit for 15 minutes. Rinse under cold water to refresh and drain. In a large bowl, combine noodles, tofu, cucumber, bell pepper, carrots, scallions, and herbs. In a separate bowl, whisk together the vinegar, soy sauce, chili flakes, and sesame oil. Pour over the noodles and toss well to combine.

Serves 4 to 6 (serving size: ⅙ recipe)

Servings of fruits and vegetables: 0.5 vegetable; **diabetes-beating phytonutrients:** phytoestrogens, genistein, quercetin, beta-sitosterol, beta-carotene

Nutrition information: 334 calories, 13 grams protein, 17 grams total fat, 2.5 grams saturated fat, no cholesterol, 32 grams carbohydrate, 2.5 grams dietary fiber, 752 milligrams sodium

Fish and Seafood

Deep sea protection! As we discussed in Chapter 4, the types of fats we eat play a big role in how our insulin functions. Fish offers heart-healthy and blood-sugar-balancing omega-3 fatty acids for real health!

❖ *Wheat Germ Encrusted Sea Bass (Full of Fiber)*

Sea bass is high in B vitamins that help reduce heart-harming homocysteine.

½ cup wheat germ
1 teaspoon freshly ground black pepper
4 tablespoons flax meal
2 4-ounce fresh sea bass fillets
Juice and zest of 1 lemon
1 tablespoon grapeseed oil or olive oil
1 teaspoon sea salt

Mix wheat germ, black pepper, and flax meal in a shallow bowl. Rinse fish. Mix lemon juice, zest, and grapeseed or olive oil. Marinate fish in mixture for 20 minutes. Season fish with sea salt and dip into flax mixture. Discard any unused mixture. Lightly spray a baking sheet pan with grapeseed oil. Broil on the middle rack for 8 minutes per side or until fish is white and flaky throughout.

Serves 2 (serving size: 1 filet)

Servings of fruits and vegetables: none; **diabetes-beating phytonutrients:** phytoestrogens, quercetin, lignin

Nutrition information: 365 calories, 32.5 grams protein, 17.5 grams total fat, 2 grams saturated fat, 47 milligrams cholesterol, 22 grams carbohydrate, 9 grams dietary fiber, 85 milligrams sodium

❖ *Salmon over Dandelion Greens with Garlic Soy Salsa (Full of Fiber)*

An omega-3 rich fish pairs up with soy for a diabetes-beating combo. Cooked and shelled edamame beans can be found in the refrigerated or frozen foods area of your supermarket. If edamame are not available, use rinsed canned cannellini beans.

2 8-ounce salmon steaks
Canola oil spray
Sea salt (optional)
4 tablespoons lemon juice
Freshly ground black pepper
1½ cups cooked edamame (soybeans)
1 cup diced tomato
½ cup chopped red onion
2 tablespoons chopped fresh parsley
1 teaspoon minced garlic
6 cups dandelion greens
1 tablespoon olive oil
Lemon wedges

Preheat oven to 350°F. Rinse salmon, lightly spray with oil, and sprinkle with sea salt if using, 2 tablespoons of lemon juice, and black pepper; refrigerate. Add beans to a nonreactive bowl and add tomato, red onion, parsley, the remaining 2 tablespoons of lemon juice, and garlic; mix well and refrigerate. Rinse dandelion greens, pat dry, and set aside. Heat large sauté pan over medium heat, add olive oil, and sauté dandelion greens until wilted. Set aside and keep warm.

Spray a baking sheet with canola oil. Place salmon on the sheet and bake for 15 minutes. Fish should be firm and opaque and flake easily. On two plates, arrange dandelion greens as bed. Lay salmon over dandelion greens, spoon garlic soybean salsa over it, and serve with lemon wedges.

Serves 2 (serving size: 1 salmon steak)

Servings of fruits and vegetables: 4.5 vegetables; **diabetes-beating phytonutrients:** quercetin, glutathione, phytoestrogens, lignin, allicin, beta-sitosterol

Nutrition information: 495 calories, 41 grams protein, 20 grams total fat, 2.5 grams saturated fat, 62 milligrams cholesterol, 40 grams carbohydrate, 14 grams dietary fiber, 230 milligrams sodium

Grilled Tuna with Mango Kiwi Salsa

Oh-megas! This delicious fish dish is paired with a tropical salsa packed with antioxidants.

1 pound fresh tuna
1 teaspoon canola oil
1 teaspoon grated fresh ginger

1 small jalapeño pepper (or to taste), seeded and chopped
¼ teaspoon sea salt (optional)
½ teaspoon freshly ground black pepper
1 tablespoon fresh lime juice
1 cup peeled and diced kiwi
¾ cup peeled and diced mango
3 tablespoons finely chopped red onion
2½ teaspoons chopped fresh cilantro
1 teaspoon fresh lemon juice
8 cups (packed) mesclun (mixed baby salad greens)

Preheat grill or broiler. Cut tuna into 16 cubes and place in a nonmetal bowl. Add oil and toss fish to coat. Add ½ teaspoon ginger, jalapeño, ⅛ teaspoon sea salt (if using), a few grinds of pepper, and lime juice. Toss to combine. Set aside while making salsa or cover and refrigerate up to 30 minutes.

In a medium bowl, add kiwi, mango, onion, remaining ginger, cilantro, remaining sea salt (if using), and lemon juice. Set aside.

String marinated tuna cubes loosely on skewers. Grill for 3 minutes. Turn and grill until fish is cooked through, 1 to 2 minutes more. (To broil, arrange fish in one layer in a shallow pan. Broil 3 minutes. Turn fish, using tongs. Broil until fish is cooked through, 1 to 2 minutes more). Divide mesclun greens among 4 plates and top with grilled tuna and salsa.

Serves 4 (serving size: 4 ounces tuna and ¼ salsa mixture, 1 plate greens)

Servings of fruits and vegetables: 1 vegetable, 1 fruit; **diabetes-beating phytonutrients:** curcumin, quercetin, beta-carotene, beta-sitosterol

Nutrition information: 200 calories, 28 grams protein, 3 grams total fat, 0.5 gram saturated fat, 53 milligrams cholesterol, 17 grams carbohydrates, 4.5 grams dietary fiber, 216 milligrams sodium

*P*an-Seared Tuna with Pineapple Vinaigrette

This vinaigrette goes really well with other grilled fish, grilled chicken, or over mixed greens salad.

1 tablespoon extra-virgin olive oil
1 garlic clove, minced
¼ cup orange juice
1 teaspoon orange zest
1 teaspoon lime or lemon zest
1 teaspoon freshly ground black pepper
2 teaspoons chopped fresh thyme
4 6-ounce tuna steaks (½-inch thick)
1 cup chopped fresh pineapple, plus slices for garnish
1 cup chopped yellow bell pepper
2 teaspoons white wine vinegar
1 tablespoon seeded and minced jalapeño pepper
½ teaspoon curry powder
½ teaspoon freshly ground black pepper
1 tablespoon sesame oil

Create marinade by combining first seven ingredients in a shallow dish. Place tuna steaks in dish, cover, and refrigerate for 1 hour. Create vinaigrette by pureeing pineapple until smooth. Add bell pepper, vinegar, jalapeño, curry, and black pepper and process until smooth, gradually adding oil. Heat nonstick skillet over high heat. Remove tuna from the marinade, and cook 2 minutes per side. Add vinaigrette to serving dishes, lay tuna steak on top, garnish with fresh pineapple slices, and serve.

Serves 4 (serving size: 1 tuna steak with garnish)

Servings of fruits and vegetables: 0.5 vegetable, 0.5 fruit; **diabetes-beating phytonutrients:** quercetin, allicin, beta-sitosterol, lignans

Nutrition information: 290 calories, 41 grams protein, 9 grams total fat, 1.5 grams saturated fat, 77 milligrams cholesterol, 10 grams carbohydrates, 1 gram dietary fiber, 65 milligrams sodium

✤ *Mustard Baked Salmon with Lentils (Full of Fiber)*

This hearty, Mediterranean-inspired meal pairs lentils with fish for a dish that's full of protein and fiber, not to mention a boatload of phytonutrients.

2 cups dried green, pink, or brown lentils, sorted and rinsed
1 cup diced carrots
½ cup diced celery
1 cup chopped leeks
½ cup chopped onion
6 whole garlic cloves
1 bay leaf
⅓ cup olive oil
2 tablespoons vinegar
¼ cup large-grain prepared mustard
4 3-ounce salmon fillets
½ cup chopped parsley

Combine lentils with carrots, celery, leeks, onion, garlic, bay leaf, and 3 tablespoons olive oil in a pot. Sauté over medium heat for 5 minutes. Add 4 cups of water and cover. Simmer 1 hour until tender. Turn off heat. Add vinegar. Preheat oven to 425°F. Blend mustard and remaining olive oil and spread mixture onto the salmon fillets. Oil a cooking rack and place it in a roasting pan. Place fillets on rack and cook for 10 minutes or until salmon is opaque and flaky. Stir parsley into lentils and divide among four plates. Place salmon atop lentils and serve.

Serves 4 (serving size: 4 oz.)

Servings of fruits and vegetables: 2 vegetables; **diabetes-beating phytonutrients:** quercetin, sulfides, kaempferol, carotenoids, lignans, phytoestrogens

Nutrition information: 466 calories, 28 grams protein, 26 grams total fat, 4 grams saturated fat, 447 milligrams cholesterol, 32 grams carbohydrate, 11 grams dietary fiber, 688 milligrams sodium

Fisherman's Stew

Soup-er for the heart! This B-vitamin-rich favorite includes tarragon for a unique flavor.

2 teaspoons extra-virgin olive oil
1 medium onion, chopped
1 small garlic clove, minced
1 cup bottled clam juice
1 medium potato, peeled and cut in ¾-inch dice
4 plum tomatoes, seeded and chopped
10 ounces fresh cod, cut into 2-inch-square pieces

6 ounces sea scallops
1 tablespoon fresh tarragon, chopped, or 1 teaspoon dried
   tarragon
½ teaspoon sea salt (optional)
½ teaspoon freshly ground black pepper

In a small Dutch oven or pot, heat oil over medium-high heat. Sauté onion and garlic until translucent, about 4 minutes. Pour in clam juice and ½ cup of water. When the liquid comes to a boil, add potatoes and tomatoes. Reduce heat to a simmer, cover, and cook 10 minutes. Add fish, scallops, and tarragon. Simmer until fish is opaque in center and flakes easily, about 4 to 5 minutes, depending on thickness. Season with sea salt (if using) and pepper and serve.

Serves 4 (serving size: 1 cup)

Servings of fruits and vegetables: 1 vegetable; **diabetes-beating phytonutrients:** allicin, glutathione, beta-sitosterol

Nutrition information: 142 calories, 21 grams protein, 3 grams total fat, 0.5 gram saturated fat, 45 milligrams cholesterol, 7 grams carbohydrate, 1 gram dietary fiber, 110 milligrams sodium

Crispy Citrus Tuna

Oranges, a low-glycemic-index food, team up with omega-3-rich tuna for a spectacular blood-sugar balancing combination.

1½ cups orange juice
2 tablespoons dry white wine
2 tablespoons cornstarch

2 large oranges, peeled and sectioned
2 tablespoons chopped fresh cilantro
2 tablespoons cornmeal
½ teaspoon sea salt
¼ teaspoon pepper
4 6-ounce tuna steaks (½ inch thick)
4 teaspoon olive oil

Whisk orange juice, wine, and cornstarch in a small saucepan until smooth. Bring to a boil over medium-high heat and cook, stirring, until sauce boils and thickens, about 2 minutes. Remove from the heat and stir in orange sections. Keep warm. Mix cilantro, cornmeal, salt, and pepper in a pie plate. Coat both sides of the tuna steaks with cornmeal mixture, pressing firmly so mixture adheres. Heat 2 teaspoons oil in a large cast-iron skillet over medium-high heat until hot, but not smoking. Sear tuna until done to taste, 2 to 3 minutes on each side for medium-rare. Add remaining oil just before turning fish. Serve with the sauce.

Serves 4 (serving size: 1 tuna steak and ¼ sauce)

Servings of fruits and vegetables: 1.5 fruits; **diabetes-beating phytonutrients:** quercetin, hesperidin

---

Nutrition information: 324 calories, 28 grams protein, 6 grams total fat, 1 gram saturated fat, 51 milligrams cholesterol, 38 grams carbohydrate, 3 grams dietary fiber, 375 milligrams sodium

---

Salmon Vegetable Pâté

This healthy dip is a perfect alternative to "chips and dip." Serve it with whole-grain crackers for a delicious hors d'oeuvre.

6 ounces fresh poached salmon, picked, or canned pink
   salmon, drained
4 ounces fat-free cream cheese, room temperature
1 tablespoon canola or soy mayonnaise
2 tablespoons fresh lemon juice
3 tablespoons finely chopped fresh dill
2 tablespoons minced red onion
½ teaspoon sea salt
Freshly ground pepper
Fresh vegetables suitable for stuffing, such as large cherry
   tomatoes, new potatoes, cucumber, radishes, or mushroom caps
Dill sprigs for garnish

In a food processor, puree salmon, cream cheese, mayon-naise, and lemon juice. Mix in dill and onion and season with salt and pepper. Use immediately or refrigerate, tightly covered, up to 24 hours. Prepare vegetables for stuffing. Cut the tops off of the tomatoes, scoop out the flesh, and cut a thin slice off of the bottom if necessary so they stand upright. Boil or steam tiny new potatoes until just tender and halve if not very small. Cut thin slice off of the bottoms so they will stand upright. Using a melon baller, scoop out about half the flesh of each potato. Cut cucum-bers in half crosswise, then into lengthwise halves or quarters, depending on size. Using tip of small spoon, create a deep groove down center, removing seeds. To stuff the vegetables, use a small pastry bag or improvise, using waxed paper rolled into cone. Pipe pâté into the cavities of vegetables, mounding to form slightly rounded tops. Garnish with small sprigs of dill on top.

Serves 6 (serving size: 2 ounces of pâté)

Servings of fruits and vegetables: none; **diabetes-beating phytonutrients:** quercetin, beta-sitosterol, anthocyanins

---

Nutrition information: 85 calories, 8 grams protein, 5 grams total fat, 1 gram saturated fat, 12 milligrams cholesterol, 2 grams carbohydrate, less than 0.5 gram dietary fiber, 230 milligrams sodium

---

*S*teamed Mussels with Saffron Sauce

A spicy dish full of protein with Mediterranean appeal, mussels deliver a good dose of heart-helping vitamin B_{12} and immune-boosting zinc.

1 large onion, chopped
2 cups fish stock or clam juice
1 cup dry white wine
¼ teaspoon saffron powder
1 tablespoon Dijon mustard
2 cloves garlic, minced
¼ cup extra-virgin olive oil
1 pound mussels, debearded
4 tablespoons fresh parsley

Sauté onion with stock and wine, simmering for 15 minutes. Whisk saffron, mustard, and garlic with oil. Thin with 1 tablespoon stock. Bring stock to a boil, add mussels and stir in 2 tablespoons mustard sauce. Cook 5 minutes, until shells open. Divide between four bowls, stir in parsley, drizzle with mustard sauce, and serve.

Serves 4 (serving size: ¼ pound mussels)

Servings of fruits and vegetables: none; **diabetes-beating phytonutrients:** lignans, quercetin, sulfides

Nutrition information: 294 calories, 17 grams protein, 18 grams total fat, 3 grams saturated fat, 33 milligrams cholesterol, 7 grams carbohydrate, less than 1 gram dietary fiber, 610 milligrams sodium

---

Sautéed Shrimp and Snow Peas with Rice Noodles

Pad thai noodles are a wider version of rice noodles, found in Asian markets.

8 ounces rice noodles (pad thai noodles or rice vermicelli)
3 tablespoons reduced-sodium soy sauce
2 tablespoons lemon juice
2 teaspoons sesame oil
1 cup white wine
½ teaspoon cornstarch
½ teaspoon black pepper
Canola oil spray
1 pound large shrimp, peeled and deveined
1 tablespoon grated fresh ginger
8 ounces snow peas
½ cup chopped scallions

Bring 1 quart of water to a boil. Pour over rice noodles and let sit for 15 minutes. Drain, refresh under cold water, and drain again. Set aside. In a small bowl, combine soy sauce, lemon juice, sesame oil, white wine, cornstarch, and black pepper. Set aside. Heat a large sauté pan or wok sprayed with canola oil. Add shrimp and stir until they start to turn pink. Add ginger and snow peas. Cook for 2 minutes. Add broth mixture and let it cook for 5 minutes, or until sauce thickens. Add noodles and toss in the sauce to combine. Let it cook in the sauce over medium heat for 2 minutes. Divide noodles with sauce among four plates; sprinkle with scallions and serve.

Serves 4 (serving size: 4 ounces shrimp and ¼ noodles and sauce)

Servings of fruits and vegetables: 0.5 vegetable; **diabetes-beating phytonutrients:** curcumin, beta-sitosterol, beta-carotene, genistein

Nutrition information: 375 calories, 30 grams protein, 1.5 grams total fat, no saturated fat, 220 milligrams cholesterol, 50 grams carbohydrate, 2 grams dietary fiber, 640 milligrams sodium

Garden Entrées

On the lighter side, these meals are a perfect example of how to give your vegetables center stage without sacrificing flavor.

✤ Pasta with Asparagus and Lemon (Full of Fiber)

A tangy pasta dish boasting glutathione and folate-rich asparagus.

13½ ounces whole-wheat spaghetti
1 large lemon
2 tablespoons unsalted butter
2 tablespoons olive oil
10 ounces asparagus, cut into 3-inch pieces
½ cup white wine
Sea salt (optional)
Freshly ground black pepper
⅓ cup freshly grated Parmesan or parmigiana-reggiano cheese
2 tablespoons chopped fresh parsley

Boil 1 gallon of water for the pasta. Cook pasta to al dente, about 8 minutes. Drain the pasta and reserve. Meanwhile, grate the zest of the lemon into a small bowl then squeeze the juice from the lemon into the same bowl. Set aside. Melt the butter in a large skillet over medium-high heat. When the butter is browned and fragrant (after about 2 minutes) add the olive oil, lemon juice, lemon zest, asparagus, and white wine. Cook for 3 minutes. Asparagus should be bright green. Add the pasta and mix well. Remove the pan from the heat and season to taste with salt (if using) and pepper. Add the cheese and toss well. Sprinkle with parsley and serve immediately.

Serves 4 (serving size: ¼ recipe)

Servings of fruits and vegetables: 0.5 vegetable; **diabetes-beating phytonutrients:** glutathione, quercetin

Nutrition information: 510 calories, 18 grams protein, 16 grams total fat, 6 grams saturated fat, 20 milligrams cholesterol, 79 grams carbohydrate, 14 grams dietary fiber, 290 milligrams sodium

Asian Tofu Cakes

Phytoestrogen-rich tofu pairs up with Asian spices to make these high protein patties.

For the cakes
2 tablespoons sesame seeds
15 ounces firm tofu, drained and rinsed
5 egg whites
⅓ cup whole-wheat flour
1 tablespoon freshly grated ginger
1 medium carrot, shredded
3 scallions, green parts only, sliced thin
⅓ cup frozen peas
1 tablespoon low-sodium soy sauce
½ teaspoon curry powder
1 garlic clove, crushed
2 teaspoons sesame oil

For the sauce
6 tablespoons low-sodium soy sauce
1 teaspoon toasted sesame oil or chili oil
1 teaspoon rice vinegar
2 teaspoons chopped scallions

In a skillet, toast sesame seeds until golden brown, about 1 minute; transfer to a plate and set aside. Mash tofu in a medium bowl with a fork to crumble. Mix in egg whites, flour, ginger, carrots, scallions, peas, soy sauce, curry powder, and minced garlic until well blended. Heat sesame oil in a large nonstick skillet. Add about ¼ cup of the tofu mixture to pan, flattening with a spatula to form cakes. Cook until golden brown, about 2 minutes per side. Repeat the process using more sesame oil until all the tofu mixture is used.

Make the sauce in a small bowl, mixing ingredients well. Serve tofu cakes sprinkled with sesame seeds and sauce on the side.

Serves 12 cakes (serving size: 2 cakes)

Servings of fruits and vegetables: 0.5 vegetable; **diabetes-beating phytonutrients:** phytoestrogens, quercetin, curcumin, genistein

Nutrition information: 160 calories, 14 grams protein, 7 grams total fat, 0.5 gram saturated fat, no cholesterol, 13 grams carbohydrate, 3 grams dietary fiber, 660 milligrams sodium

✤ *Stuffed Eggplant with Peanut Sauce (Full of Fiber)*

The purple color of eggplant comes from anthocyanins that help to protect the heart and blood vessels. The red onions add a sweet flavor plus quercetin. The small size of these Japanese eggplants makes them perfect for this delicious dish.

> 2 Japanese eggplants (4 ounces each)
> Canola oil spray
> 1 cup diced red onions
> ¾ cup diced red bell pepper
> 1 cup bias-sliced snow peas
> 2 tablespoons low-sodium chicken broth
> 2 tablespoons low-sodium soy sauce
> 1 tablespoon hoisin sauce
> 1 tablespoon creamy natural peanut butter
> 1 teaspoon grated ginger
> 1 teaspoon minced garlic
> 1 cup diced bok choy
> 1 cup shredded carrots
> 1 cup hot cooked rice (basmati or brown)

Preheat oven to 350°F. Halve each eggplant. On a baking sheet that has been sprayed with canola oil, place the eggplant halves flesh side down and bake for about 6 minutes or until they start to soften. Using a melon baller, scoop out the flesh, leaving ¼-inch-thick shells. Chop the eggplant flesh and set aside. In a medium sauté pan sprayed with canola oil, and add the onions, peppers, and chopped eggplant. Stir. Add snow peas and chicken broth. Cook for 2 minutes or until snow peas turn bright green. Remove from the heat and set aside. In a separate bowl, combine soy sauce, hoisin sauce, peanut butter, ginger, and garlic. Mix well. Add sautéed vegetables, bok choy, carrots, and cooked rice. Mix well and mound into the eggplant shells. Arrange the eggplant shells side by side in a casserole dish. Cover with aluminum foil and bake for 10 minutes or until all are heated through.

Serves 2 (serving size: 2 filled eggplant halves)

Servings of fruits and vegetables: 8.5 vegetables; **diabetes-beating phytonutrients:** quercetin, beta-carotene, genistein, curcumin

---

Nutrition information: 410 calories, 15 grams protein, 6 grams total fat, 1 gram saturated fat, no cholesterol, 81 grams carbohydrate, 20 grams dietary fiber, 770 milligrams sodium

---

Vegetable Lettuce Rolls

A mainstay in Asian cultures, these lettuce envelopes cradle a colorful array of veggies that pack an antioxidant round kick! Date sugar is available in health-food stores and gourmet markets.

3 to 4 ounces thin rice noodles
8 large leaves green leaf lettuce
2 scallions, green part only, cut in 3-inch pieces
1 medium carrot, peeled and julienned
3-inch-long piece of seedless cucumber, peeled and
    julienned
½ cup (loosely packed) julienned basil leaves
½ red bell pepper, cut in thin strips
24 fresh cilantro leaves, washed and dried
½ cup (loosely packed) thinly sliced mint leaves
1 shallot, minced very fine
⅛ teaspoon red pepper flakes
2 tablespoons low-sodium soy sauce

2 tablespoons rice vinegar
1 teaspoon date sugar

Bring 3 cups of water to a boil and pour over the rice noodles. Let it sit for 15 minutes. Drain, refresh under cold water,
and drain well. Use scissors to cut noodles into 3-inch lengths.
Arrange lettuce on a serving platter. Arrange julienned scallions,
carrots, and cucumbers in separate mounds on a second platter.
Add red pepper, cilantro, and mint leaves, mounded into separate
piles. In medium bowl, mix together shallot, pepper flakes, soy
sauce, rice vinegar, date sugar, and ¼ cup of cold water. Set aside.

On each leaf, place about 2 ounces of noodles and a combination of all the vegetables. Roll the leaf securing it like a wrap.
Repeat with all the other leaves. Serve with the sauce on the side.

Serves 4 (serving size: 2 rolls)

Servings of fruits and vegetables: 1.5 vegetables; **diabetes-beating
phytonutrients:** beta-sitosterol, beta-carotene, quercetin, tannins

---

Nutrition information: 160 calories, 3 grams protein, 0.5 gram total
fat, no saturated fat, no cholesterol, 35 grams carbohydrate, 3 grams
dietary fiber, 340 milligrams sodium

Vegetable Frittata

*Eggs-ellent! High-protein eggs team up with a variety of veggies to
lay on the phytonutrient protection.*

1 12-ounce baking potato, peeled and cut into chunks
3 large eggs

3 large egg whites
3 ounces fresh spinach (3 loosely packed cups), steamed
  and chopped
3 medium or 2 large whole scallions, chopped
½ cup chopped cilantro
½ cup seeded and diced tomatoes
1 jalapeño or other chili pepper, seeded and chopped
  (optional)
½ teaspoon ground turmeric
½ teaspoon sea salt
¼ teaspoon freshly ground black pepper
Canola oil spray

In a large saucepan, cover potato with cold water. Bring to a boil over medium-high heat. Reduce heat and cook until potato is soft when pierced through with a knife, about 20 minutes. Beat eggs and whites together in a medium bowl. Drain potato and lightly mash. Add mashed potato to eggs. Add spinach, scallions, cilantro, tomato, chili pepper (if using), turmeric, salt, and pepper. Mix with a rubber spatula until ingredients are well combined.

Coat a medium, nonstick skillet generously with canola cooking spray. Set pan over medium-high heat. Add egg mixture, spreading it into an even layer. Cover pan and reduce heat to medium. Cook until frittata is puffed, browned on the bottom, and the center is lightly set, about 10 minutes. Remove pan from heat. Invert pan, releasing the frittata onto a large dinner plate. Place the pan back on the stove and slide the frittata, browned side up, back into the pan. Cook uncovered until bottom browns, 4 to 5 minutes. Slide frittata onto a serving plate and let sit 5 minutes. Cut into wedges and serve hot or at room temperature.

Serves 4 (serving size: ¼ frittata)

Servings of fruits and vegetables: 0.5 vegetable; **diabetes-beating phytonutrients:** beta-carotene, beta-sitosterol, quercetin, saponins, lycopene

Nutrition information: 150 calories, 10 grams protein, 4.5 grams total fat, 1.5 grams saturated fat, 160 milligrams cholesterol, 19 grams carbohydrate, 3 grams dietary fiber, 420 milligrams sodium

*M*editerranean Spinach Pie

A healthier version of the Greek spanakopita, lutein-rich spinach helps protect eyesight, a common complication of diabetes.

1 10-ounce bag fresh spinach
Canola oil spray
2 tablespoons nonhydrogenated bread crumbs
1 tablespoon wheat germ
3 egg whites
3 large eggs
½ cup crumbled feta cheese
½ cup fat-free half and half
1 cup low-fat ricotta cheese
2 cloves garlic, crushed
½ cup seeded and diced tomatoes
1 teaspoon sea salt (optional)
Freshly ground black pepper
Pinch of freshly grated nutmeg

Preheat oven to 350°F. In a medium sauté pan, bring ½ cup water to a simmer. Add spinach and cook until it is all wilted. Cool, squeeze out liquid, and chop. Lightly coat a 9-inch pie dish with canola oil spray. Sprinkle 1 tablespoon bread crumbs and wheat germ inside the pan to coat. In a bowl, beat the remaining ingredients together and add in spinach. Pour mixture into pie pan, smooth it out, and bake for 35 minutes or until top is light golden and slightly puffed. Let stand 10 minutes; slice into 4 wedges and serve.

Serves 4 (serving size: 1 wedge)

Servings of fruits and vegetables: 0.75 vegetable; **diabetes-beating phytonutrients:** saponins, allicin, beta-sitosterol, glutathione

Nutrition information: 220 calories, 19 grams protein, 11 grams total fat, 6 grams saturated fat, 190 milligrams cholesterol, 12 grams carbohydrate, 3 grams dietary fiber, 460 milligrams sodium

✣ *Tempeh Cacciatore (Full of Fiber)*

Meatless wonder! Tempeh has a meaty, nutty texture, and as a soy product, it helps protect the heart. Serve this on a bed of whole-grain spaghetti or brown rice.

1 cup thinly sliced onion
½ cup chopped green bell pepper
2 tablespoons olive oil
1 clove garlic, minced
1 cup sliced fresh mushrooms
8 ounces tempeh, cubed
⅓ cup vegetable broth
2½ cups peeled and chopped tomatoes
⅓ cup red wine

1 bay leaf
2 teaspoons low-sodium soy sauce
½ teaspoon dry thyme
½ teaspoon oregano
1 teaspoon basil

Sauté onion and green pepper in olive oil over low heat until onion is translucent. Stir in garlic, mushrooms, and tempeh. Cook another 5 minutes or so. Add vegetable broth, tomatoes, wine, bay leaf, soy sauce, thyme, oregano, and basil and bring to a boil. Reduce heat and simmer for 30 minutes stirring from time to time.

Serves 4 (serving size: ¼ mixture)

Servings of fruits and vegetables: 2.0 vegetables; **diabetes-beating phytonutrients:** phytoestrogens, genistein, quercetin, glutathione, flavonols

Nutrition information: 250 calories, 15 grams protein, 12 grams total fat, 1.5 grams saturated fat, no cholesterol, 21 grams carbohydrate, 7 grams dietary fiber, 140 milligrams sodium

Risotto Tart with Tomatoes, Onions, and Peppers

This delicious tart uses rice as the crust. Layered with veggies, this healthy alternative to pizza is sure to please.

Vegetable oil spray
1 tablespoon olive oil
1 cup chopped onion

1 cup seeded and chopped green bell pepper

3 garlic cloves, minced

2 cups chopped fresh plum tomatoes

2 tablespoons chopped fresh basil

1½ teaspoons fresh thyme leaves

2 teaspoons sea salt (optional)

½ teaspoon freshly ground pepper

3 cups cooked arborio rice (start with 1½ cups raw rice, as it will double after cooked)

1 egg white

1 cup shredded reduced-fat mozzarella cheese

1 tablespoon grated Romano cheese

Preheat oven to 400°F. Coat an 11-inch pizza pan or cookie sheet with cooking spray. Heat oil in a medium skillet over medium-high heat. Sauté onions, green pepper, and garlic until soft, about 4 minutes. Add tomatoes. Cook, stirring occasionally until liquid has evaporated from tomatoes, about 12 minutes. Stir in 1 tablespoon basil and 1 teaspoon thyme. Season with 1 teaspoon sea salt (if using) and ¼ teaspoon pepper, or to taste. Combine rice with egg white, remaining basil and thyme, and remaining salt (if using) and pepper. Mound rice in the center of prepared pan. Cover rice with plastic wrap.

Using your fingers, pat and shape rice into a 10½-inch circle, about ½ inch thick, making a rim around the edge. Lift away the wrap. Sprinkle half the mozzarella cheese over rice. Cover cheese with cooked tomato mixture. Top with remaining mozzarella. Sprinkle Romano cheese over the top. Bake until cheese is bubbly and edge of rice crust is crisp, 15 to 18 minutes. Serve hot.

Serves 4 (serving size: ¼ tart)

Servings of fruits and vegetables: 1.5 vegetables; **diabetes-beating phytonutrients:** beta-sitosterol, lignin, glutathione

Nutrition information: 280 calories, 13 grams protein, 8 grams total fat, 2.5 grams saturated fat, 10 milligrams cholesterol, 38 grams carbohydrate, 3 grams dietary fiber, 230 milligrams sodium

❖ *Vegetarian Paella (Full of Fiber)*

A hearty vegetable stew flavored with saffron, onions, and garlic. This creative concoction helps keep blood sugar on an even keel with phytonutrients like quercetin and beta-sitosterol.

14 ounces vegetable stock, plus more if needed
1 teaspoon saffron
2 tablespoons olive oil
1½ cups finely chopped onion
2 garlic cloves, crushed
2 Jerusalem artichokes, diced (optional)
1 eggplant, diced (about 3 cups)
2 cups combination diced red, yellow, and green
    bell peppers
1 cup sliced celery stalks
1 teaspoon Spanish paprika
1 cup Spanish short-grain rice
¼ cup dry white wine
1½ cups canned crushed tomatoes
½ cup diced green beans
2 tablespoons sliced pitted black olives
½ cup frozen peas
2 tablespoons chopped flat-leaf parsley
Lemon wedges for garnish

Put vegetable stock and the saffron in a large pot and bring to a boil. Remove from heat and set aside. Heat the oil in a large pan and cook the onion and garlic for 5 minutes over medium heat, until golden. Add the artichokes (if using), eggplant, bell peppers, celery, paprika, and rice and stir to coat in the oil. Cook for 2 to 3 minutes, stirring occasionally, until the rice becomes transparent. Pour in the wine and saffron-infused stock. Stir in the tomatoes, reduce the heat, and cook for 20 minutes, until tender. Stir in the green beans, olives, and peas. Add more stock if the rice is not cooked. Let it sit covered for 5 minutes. Garnish with parsley and place the lemon wedges on the side.

Serves 4 (serving size: ¼ paella mixture)

Servings of fruits and vegetables: 6.5 vegetables; **diabetes-beating phytonutrients:** beta-carotene, beta-sitosterol, quercetin

Nutrition information: 430 calories, 12 grams protein, 10 grams total fat, 1.5 grams saturated fat, no cholesterol, 80 grams carbohydrates, 15 grams dietary fiber, 630 milligrams sodium

---

❖ *Penne with Portobello and Veggie Sausage (Full of Fiber)*

Soy is a healthy stand-in for meat sausage and goes well with the rich flavor of portly portobello mushrooms.

1 tablespoon canola or extra-virgin olive oil
1 cup chopped onion
2 cloves garlic, crushed
1 14-ounce package veggie sausage

1 cup reduced-sodium vegetable broth
1 28-ounce can no-salt-added crushed or whole tomatoes
1 large portobello mushroom, sliced (about 2½ cups)
½ cup sliced black olives
½ cup chopped combination of fresh herbs: basil, oregano,
   and parsley
2 teaspoons sea salt
Freshly ground black pepper
1 12-ounce box whole-grain pasta
½ cup parmigiana-reggiano cheese, grated

In a large sauté pan, heat oil and sauté onion and garlic. Add veggie sausage stirring constantly to break up. When all veggie sausage is crumbled and browned, add broth, tomatoes, portobello mushrooms, olives, and herbs. Simmer for 20 minutes stirring from time to time. Season with 1 teaspoon sea salt and ground black pepper, if desired.

Meanwhile, bring 1 gallon of water to a boil. Add 1 teaspoon of sea salt. Add pasta and cook until al dente, about 10 minutes. Drain. Toss pasta with the sausage portobello sauce, sprinkle with parmigiana-reggiano cheese, and serve.

Serves 6 (serving size: ⅙ pasta mixture)

Servings of fruits and vegetables: 1.5 vegetables; **diabetes-beating phytonutrients:** genistein, phytoestrogens, allicin, beta-sitosterol, glutathione, quercetin, beta-carotene

---

Nutrition information: 380 calories, 24 grams protein, 7 grams total fat, 1.5 grams saturated fat, 5 milligrams cholesterol, 62 grams carbohydrate, 11 grams dietary fiber, 580 milligrams sodium

---

Chicken and Turkey

Poultry provides a bevy of B vitamins that help to reduce levels of heart-harming homocysteine, while delivering a good source of blood-sugar-balancing protein.

Pasta with Chicken and Veggies

Asparagus, peas, and tomatoes team up with chicken for a colorful and healthy pasta meal.

8 ounces fresh or dried angel hair pasta
Olive oil cooking spray
1 small red onion, chopped fine (about 1 cup)
8 medium asparagus, cut in ½-inch slices
1 pound skinless, boneless chicken breast, cut into strips
½ cup frozen baby green peas
1 cup nonfat, reduced-sodium chicken broth
12 cherry tomatoes, halved
Sea salt
Freshly ground black pepper
½ cup (2 ounces) crumbled feta cheese
1 tablespoon extra-virgin olive oil
¼ cup chopped fresh basil leaves
¼ cup chopped fresh flat-leaf parsley

Cook pasta in ½ gallon of boiling water for about 7 minutes, or until al dente. Drain and set aside. Heat a large saucepan over medium-high heat and spray with oil. Sauté onion 1 minute. Add asparagus, chicken, and peas. Stir to blend. Add broth and cook until asparagus is crisp-tender, about 2 minutes. Stir in tomatoes and cook until heated through. Season to taste with sea salt and pepper. Stir in cooked pasta. Sprinkle feta cheese and extra-virgin olive oil over the top. Add basil and parsley for garnish and serve.

Serves 4 (serving size: 4 ounces chicken, ¼ pasta, ¼ vegetable mixture)

Servings of fruits and vegetables: 1 vegetable; **diabetes-beating phytonutrients:** beta-sitosterol, glutathione, genistein, quercetin

Nutrition information: 482 calories, 40 grams protein, 14 grams total fat, 4.5 grams saturated fat, 83 milligrams cholesterol, 50 grams carbohydrate, 4.5 grams dietary fiber, 430 milligrams sodium

Chicken Jambalaya

Spicy protection! Cloves and bay leaves help to balance blood sugar and give this Bayou staple authentic flavor.

1 tablespoon olive oil
1 medium onion, chopped
3 garlic cloves, minced
12 ounces skinless, boneless chicken breasts, cut into ¾-inch pieces
1 14½-ounce can whole plum tomatoes in juice, chopped
½ cup celery, cut into ½-inch slices
½ cup chopped green bell pepper
1 scallion, chopped
1 tablespoon tomato paste
1 bay leaf
1 teaspoon dried thyme
1 tablespoon chopped fresh parsley

¼ teaspoon dried red pepper flakes
1 pinch ground cloves
1 teaspoon sea salt
½ teaspoon ground black pepper
1 cup cooked, hot long-grain brown rice

In 3-quart Dutch oven, heat oil over medium-high heat. Add onion and garlic. Sauté, stirring frequently, until onion is tender but not brown, about 4 minutes. Add chicken and cook, stirring, until pieces are white on all sides. Add tomatoes with liquid. Mix in celery, bell peppers, scallion, and tomato paste. Stir in bay leaf, thyme, parsley, pepper flakes, cloves, salt, and pepper. Bring to a boil, then reduce heat and simmer until chicken is cooked and sauce has thickened, about 20 minutes. Remove bay leaf. Stir rice into chicken mixture until well combined.

Serves 4 (serving size: ¼ jambalaya recipe)

Servings of fruits and vegetables: 2 vegetables; **diabetes-beating phytonutrients:** lignin, kaempferol, beta-sitosterol, allicin, beta-carotene

Nutrition information: 223 calories, 20 grams protein, 6 grams total fat, 1 gram saturated fat, 47 milligrams cholesterol, 22 grams carbohydrate, 3.5 grams dietary fiber, 675 milligrams sodium

Chicken and Orange Stir-Fry with Rice Noodles

Wok this way! Stir-frying is a great way to keep your veggies crisp and to add flavor without adding extra calories from fat.

8 ounces rice noodles
1 tablespoon sesame seeds
Nonstick cooking spray
1 to 2 cloves garlic, minced
1 tablespoon fresh ginger or turmeric, grated
1 cup chopped green onion
1½ cups sliced mushrooms
1 cup asparagus, cut in 1-inch pieces
10 ounces cooked chicken breast
3 tablespoons low-sodium chicken broth
2 tablespoons low-sodium soy sauce
1 teaspoon cornstarch
½ cup orange juice
1 tablespoon sesame oil
1 orange, peeled, seeded, and chopped

In a medium saucepan, bring 5 cups of water to a boil. Pour over rice noodles and let it sit for 15 minutes. Drain, refresh under cold water. Set aside. Heat a small, nonstick pan over high heat. Add sesame seeds and stir constantly until seeds turn golden; transfer to a dish to cool. Set aside. Coat a large nonstick skillet lightly with cooking spray and place over medium heat. Sauté garlic and ginger or turmeric until lightly colored, about 1 minute. Add green onion and mushrooms and sauté about 2 minutes more. Add asparagus, cooked chicken, and chicken broth. Let it cook for 2 minutes. In a small bowl, combine soy sauce, cornstarch, orange juice, and sesame oil. Add to the pan, stir, and cook until vegetables are tender and sauce is thick, about 1 to 2 minutes. Toss noodles and orange pieces in with vegetables. Sprinkle with sesame seeds and serve.

Serves 4 (serving size: ¼ pasta with ¼ chicken and vegetable mixture)

Servings of fruits and vegetables: 1.0 vegetable, 0.5 fruit; **diabetes-beating phytonutrients:** curcumin, beta-carotene, quercetin, kaempferol, allicin

Nutrition information: 430 calories, 28 grams protein, 8 grams total fat, 1.5 grams saturated fat, 60 milligrams cholesterol, 61 grams carbohydrates, 4 grams dietary fiber, 460 milligrams sodium

❖ *Spicy Turkey Meatloaf with Spinach (Full of Fiber)*

A better-for-you alternative, this meatloaf doesn't lose its homestyle appeal.

½ cup rolled oats (not quick-cooking or instant)
2 egg whites, beaten until frothy
1 cup seeded and chopped tomatoes
1¼ pounds ground turkey, 93 percent lean
1½ tablespoons chili powder
2 teaspoons oregano
2 teaspoons minced garlic
¼ cup chili sauce or ketchup
Sea salt (optional)
¼ teaspoon freshly ground pepper
1 10-ounce package defrosted frozen spinach, squeezed
½ cup frozen, canned, or fresh corn kernels
Nonstick cooking spray

Preheat oven to 375°F. In a large bowl, using a fork, mix together oats, egg whites, and tomatoes. Blend in turkey, chili powder, oregano, garlic, chili sauce or ketchup, sea salt, and pepper. Mix in spinach and corn. Pack mixture firmly into a 9″ × 5″-

inch loaf pan that has been lightly coated with cooking oil spray. Bake uncovered for 45 minutes or until juices run clear when meatloaf is pierced with a knife, or internal temperature registers 165°F. Remove from oven and let meatloaf sit at least 15 minutes before serving.

Serves 4 to 6 (serving size: ⅙ of loaf)

Servings of fruits and vegetables: 1 vegetable; **diabetes-beating phytonutrients:** glutathione, quercetin, beta-sitosterol, lignan, saponins

Nutrition information: 220 calories, 24 grams protein, 7 grams total fat, 2 grams saturated fat, 55 milligrams cholesterol, 16 gram carbohydrates, 5 grams dietary fiber, 310 milligrams sodium

ʃpanish Rice and Chicken Casserole

If making this dish with the instant parboiled brown rice, cut the baking time to 30 minutes.

1 tablespoon extra-virgin olive oil
1 medium onion, chopped
1 teaspoon minced garlic
1¼ cups long-grain brown rice
1 14½-ounce can stewed tomatoes with juices
1½ cups canned low-sodium chicken broth
1 teaspoon paprika
½ teaspoon dried oregano
1 7-ounce jar roasted red peppers, drained and chopped
2 medium (about 1¼ pounds), skinless, boneless chicken breasts, diced

1 teaspoon sea salt (optional)
½ teaspoon freshly ground black pepper
1½ teaspoons dried parsley
1 bay leaf
½ cup frozen green peas

Preheat oven to 375°F. In a large sauté pan, heat the olive oil and sauté onion and garlic until translucent and fragrant. In a 2-quart casserole, combine rice, onion and garlic mixture, tomatoes, broth, paprika, oregano, roasted peppers, chicken, sea salt, pepper, parsley, and bay leaf. Cover casserole and bake 1½ hours. Stir in peas. Bake until rice is tender and chicken is cooked through. Remove bay leaf and serve.

Serves 6 to 8 (serving size: ⅛ of casserole)

Servings of fruits and vegetables: 1 vegetable; **diabetes-beating phytonutrients:** quercetin, lignan

Nutrition information: 240 calories, 19 grams protein, 4.5 grams total fat, 1 gram saturated fat, 40 milligrams cholesterol, 31 grams carbohydrate, 3 grams dietary fiber, 230 milligrams sodium

❖ *Chicken Tomatillo Enchilada (Full of Fiber)*

Queso fresco is a Mexican fresh white cheese. It can be found in the dairy cooler of your supermarket, or you can substitute fresh mozzarella cheese.

For the sauce
1 pound tomatillos, husked and rinsed
3 ounces onion

3 whole garlic cloves
½ jalapeño pepper
½ teaspoon sea salt (optional)
1 cup fresh cilantro
For the filling
14 ounces chicken broth
20 ounces skinless, boneless chicken breast
8 ounces queso fresco, crumbled
4 ounces Monterey Jack cheese, shredded
8 8-inch whole-wheat flour tortillas (taco size)
1 Hass avocado, chopped
Vegetable oil spray

To make the sauce, combine tomatillo, onion, garlic, jalapeño, and 6 cups of water. Bring to a boil. As soon as it starts to boil, remove from the heat and drain. Transfer to a blender and add sea salt (if using) and cilantro. Puree until liquefied. Set aside.

In large saucepan, bring broth to a boil. Add chicken breast and simmer for 20 minutes. Strain, and reserve broth for another use. When chicken is cool enough to handle, shred it to pieces. Set aside. Preheat oven to 350°F. Combine shredded chicken with 2½ cups of tomatillo sauce, queso fresco, and half of Monterey Jack cheese.

On each tortilla, place about ¾ cup of the chicken mixture and some chopped avocado. Roll the tortilla securing the filling like a wrap. Place rolled tortilla in a baking dish that has been lightly sprayed with vegetable oil. Repeat with the remaining tortillas.

Pour the remaining tomatillo sauce over the enchiladas, sprinkle remaining Monterey Jack cheese, and bake for 20 minutes or until golden.

Serves 6 (serving size: 1 enchilada with sauce)

Servings of fruits and vegetables: 1 vegetable; **diabetes-beating phytonutrients:** beta-carotene, beta-sitosterol, allicin, lignan, glutathione

Nutrition information: 310 calories, 26 grams protein, 13 grams total fat, 5 grams saturated fat, 60 milligrams cholesterol, 29 grams carbohydrate, 5 grams dietary fiber, 590 milligrams sodium

✥ *Corn, Zucchini, and Chicken Quesadilla (Full of Fiber)*

Whole-grain tortillas paired with veggies give Mexican food a good wrap! This is a great brunch dish that also works well for picnics. It can be served hot or at room temperature.

For the salsa
1 cup diced Roma tomatoes
1 tablespoon chopped and seeded jalapeño
2 tablespoons chopped fresh cilantro
Juice of 1 lime
1 tablespoon olive oil
For the quesadillas
1 pound cooked chicken breast, shredded
2 cups seeded and thinly sliced zucchini
½ cup corn kernels
½ cup thinly sliced red bell pepper
2 tablespoons chopped red onion
1½ teaspoons sea salt (optional)
1½ cup reduced-fat Monterey Jack cheese, grated
8 8-inch whole-wheat tortillas
Vegetable oil spray

Preheat oven to 350°F. Make the salsa by combining all the ingredients and set aside. In a medium bowl, combine chicken, zucchini, corn, bell pepper, red onion, sea salt (if using), and cheese. Mix well to combine. Spread one fourth of the mixture on a tortilla, being sure to cover the whole surface. Sprinkle about 2 tablespoons of salsa over it. Place another tortilla on top and transfer to a baking sheet pan lightly sprayed with vegetable oil. Repeat with the remaining tortillas. Bake the quesadillas for 15 minutes or until cheese is all melted and golden. Serve with salsa.

Serves 4 (serving size: 1 quesadilla with ⅓ cup salsa)

Servings of fruits and vegetables: 1 vegetable; **diabetes-beating phytonutrients:** flavonoids, beta-carotene, beta-sitosterol

Nutrition information: 570 calories, 54 grams protein, 18 grams total fat, 8 grams saturated fat, 125 milligrams cholesterol, 52 grams carbohydrate, 6 grams dietary fiber, 800 milligrams sodium

Turkey, Avocado, and Tomato Tostadas

Avocados, loaded with sugar-balancing monounsaturated fats, lend a delicious creaminess to this crunchy dish.

1 tablespoon olive oil
20 ounces ground turkey, 93 percent lean
¾ cup chopped onion
3 garlic cloves, minced
1 teaspoon dried oregano

1 tablespoon chopped fresh cilantro
1 teaspoon ground cumin
½ teaspoon dried chili flakes
1 teaspoon sea salt (optional)
1 cup seeded and chopped tomatoes
6 crispy taco shells or 6-inch corn tostada
   (nonhydrogenated)
1 avocado, chopped
8 ounces queso fresco or fresh mozzarella

In a large sauté pan, heat the olive oil. Add ground turkey and cook stirring until it starts to brown, about 8 minutes. Add onion, garlic, herbs, cumin, chili flakes, and sea salt (if using). Cook until most of the liquid has evaporated. Add tomatoes and stir to combine.

Place each taco shell or tostada on a plate and top with ground turkey mixture. Sprinkle with avocado and queso fresco or mozzarella and serve immediately.

Serves 6 (serving size: 1 filled taco or tostada with approximately 1¼ ounces cheese)

Servings of fruits and vegetables: 0.5 vegetable; **diabetes-beating phytonutrients:** glutathione, quercetin, beta-sitosterol, allicin, curcumin

Nutrition information: 340 calories, 23 grams protein, 21 grams total fat, 5 grams saturated fat, 185 milligrams cholesterol, 15 grams carbohydrate, 4 grams dietary fiber, 190 milligrams sodium

❖ *Lebanese Turkey Kibbe with Tahini Sauce (Full of Fiber)*

Whole-grain bulgur is the nutritional standout star in this Lebanese dish packed with antioxidant-rich herbs. A perfect accompaniment to this dish would be a mixed green salad.

For the kibbe
20 ounces ground turkey, 93 percent lean
1¼ cups bulgur wheat
3 green onions, chopped
5 tablespoons lemon juice
1½ tablespoons olive oil
2 tablespoons chopped fresh parsley
1 tablespoon chopped fresh mint
2 teaspoons dry oregano
1 pinch cayenne pepper
1 tablespoon ground cumin
1 teaspoon sea salt (optional)
1 teaspoon freshly ground black pepper
Vegetable oil spray
For the sauce
2 tablespoons tahini
3 tablespoons lemon juice
3 tablespoons olive oil
1 teaspoon minced garlic
6 sprigs fresh parsley
1 teaspoon sea salt (optional)
1 teaspoon freshly ground black pepper

Preheat oven to 350°F. In a large bowl, combine all the kibbe ingredients, except for vegetable oil spray. Mix well to combine. Transfer to an 8-inch square pan that has been sprayed with vegetable oil. Bake for approximately 45 minutes or until it looks golden brown on the top.

While kibbee is baking, make the sauce by combining all the ingredients in a blender and ¾ cup of water and process until smooth. Serve the kibbee hot with the sauce on the side.

Serves 4 to 6 (serving size: ⅙ of recipe)

Servings of fruits and vegetables: 0.5 vegetable; **diabetes-beating phytonutrients:** quercetin, curcumin

Nutrition information: 370 calories, 20 grams protein, 21 grams total fat, 4 grams saturated fat, 65 milligrams cholesterol, 27 grams carbohydrate, 7 grams dietary fiber, 90 milligrams sodium

---

Cornish Hens with Wild Rice

A traditional chicken dish paired with low-GI rice and veggies for a unique twist on an old comfort food. Serve accompanied by cooked vegetables.

3 cups fat-free, reduced-sodium chicken broth
½ cup wild rice rinsed well
½ cup brown rice
1 teaspoon fresh or ½ teaspoon dried tarragon
Sea salt (optional)
Freshly ground pepper (optional)
2 teaspoons olive oil
½ medium onion, chopped fine
4 ounces mushrooms, sliced thin

¼ cup blanched almonds, slivered
2 Cornish hens
4 tablespoons Seville orange or regular orange marmalade

In large saucepan, bring broth to boil. Add both rices and tarragon. Bring to boil, reduce heat, cover, and simmer 45 minutes or until rice is tender. Transfer cooked rice to bowl. Season with sea salt and pepper to taste, if desired. While rice cooks, heat oil in a nonstick pan over medium heat. Add onions and sauté until soft and translucent. Raise heat to high and add mushrooms and almonds. Sauté, stirring constantly to prevent burning, about 3 minutes or until nuts are golden. Combine mixture with cooked rice. Preheat oven to 375°F. Rinse hens and trim excess fat. Season cavities with salt and pepper, then stuff with rice mixture. Season skin with salt and pepper, if desired. Place hens on rack in shallow roasting pan, breast side up. Roast hens for about 75 minutes. (Juices run clear when thigh is pricked with fork.)

Meanwhile, melt marmalade in microwave, then pour over hens to glaze during last 30 minutes of roasting. When hens are done, remove and let rest 15 minutes. Cut each hen in half, lengthwise and remove skin. Divide stuffing between four plates. Place a half of a hen on top of each bed of rice.

Serves 4 (serving size: ½ hen with ¼ stuffing mixture)

Servings of fruits and vegetables: 0.5 vegetable; **diabetes-beating phytonutrients:** quercetin, isoflavones, beta-carotene, beta-sitosterol

---

Nutrition information: 470 calories, 38 grams protein, 13 grams total fat, 2.5 grams saturated fat, 140 milligrams cholesterol, 50 grams carbohydrate, 4 grams dietary fiber, 210 milligrams sodium

Desserts and Drinks

Who says dessert can't be healthy? Try our smoothies, muffins, and other desserts to please your palette without guilt.

*P*each Flax Smoothie

Give it a whirl! Flavonoids from the peaches get mixed up with omega-3 rich flaxseed.

½ cup plain reduced-fat yogurt
1 cup frozen, unsweetened peaches, chopped or sliced
2 tablespoons frozen apple juice concentrate
½ teaspoon flaxseed oil

Combine all the ingredients in a blender. Blend until smooth.

Serves: 2 (serving size: 6 fluid ounces)

Servings of fruits and vegetables: 1.25 fruit; **diabetes-beating phytonutrients:** lignans

Nutrition information: 180 calories, 9 grams protein, 4 grams total fat, 1 gram saturated fat, 5 milligrams cholesterol, 30 grams carbohydrate, 3 grams dietary fiber, 95 milligrams sodium

Strawberry Banana Smoothie

The tofu adds silkiness and stabilizing phytoestrogens to the berry blend.

1 cup fresh strawberries, quartered
½ cup light vanilla soy milk
⅓ cup soft silken tofu
1 frozen banana, sliced
2 tablespoons frozen apple juice concentrate

Combine the strawberries, soy milk, and tofu in a blender. Add the banana and apple juice concentrate. Blend until smooth.

Serves 2 (serving size: 6 fluid ounces)

Servings of fruits and vegetables: 1.5 fruits; **diabetes-beating phytonutrients:** beta-carotene, flavonoids, glutathione, genistein, phytoestrogens

Nutrition information: 160 calories, 5 grams protein, 2.5 grams total fat, no saturated fat, no cholesterol, 32 grams carbohydrate, 3 grams dietary fiber, 40 milligrams sodium

❖ Chocolate Mint Berry Smoothie (Full of Fiber)

Have your chocolate and drink it, too! The berries, mint, and cocoa in this smoothie provide antioxidant phytonutrients and heavenly taste. Grab a straw and try it for dessert tonight.

¾ cup chocolate soy milk
1¼ cups frozen, unsweetened raspberries
½ medium banana, sliced
¾ cup chocolate sorbet
2 tablespoons fresh mint, chopped

Combine the soy milk, raspberries, and banana in a blender. Add the sorbet and mint. Blend until smooth.

Serves 2 (serving size: 5 fluid ounces)

Servings of fruits and vegetables: 1 fruit; **diabetes-beating phytonutrients:** phytoestrogens, genistein, flavonols, glutathione

Nutrition information: 200 calories, 5 grams protein, 2.5 grams total fat, no saturated fat, no cholesterol, 43 grams carbohydrate, 9 grams dietary fiber, 65 milligrams sodium

Spiced Chai

Thanks to its unique mix of spices, frangrant chai is a wonderful blood-sugar balancer. You can omit the soy milk and the calories will be negligible.

4 cardamom pods
4-inch cinnamon stick
4 cloves
8 whole black peppercorns
1 vanilla bean, split in half lengthwise
1 inch fresh ginger, peeled
4 teaspoons black tea or 4 teabags

2 cups 2 percent milk or plain soy milk
1 tablespoon honey

Place cardamom, cinnamon stick, cloves, peppercorns, and vanilla bean in a saucepan. Add 2 cups water. Using the finest holes on a grater, grate ginger over pot to catch all the ginger juices. Bring to a boil over medium-high heat. Reduce heat and simmer gently 3 minutes. Add tea, cover pot, and remove from heat. Steep spices for 10 minutes. Remove vanilla bean and scrape seeds into the liquid. Return pot to medium-high heat and bring back to a boil, uncovered. Add milk. When mixture is about to boil again, stir in honey, strain chai, and pour into mugs to serve.

Serves 4 (serving size: 8 fluid ounces)

Servings of fruits and vegetables: none; **diabetes-beating phytonutrients:** tannins, curcumin, phytoestrogens, genistein, catechins

---

Nutrition information: 80 calories, 4 grams protein, 2.5 grams total fat, 1.5 grams saturated fat, 10 milligrams cholesterol, 10 grams carbohydrate, no dietary fiber, 50 milligrams sodium

---

Gingered Green Tea Cooler

Teas to ease diabetes! Long revered for their beneficial effects on insulin function and action as antioxidants, this is a drink for your health.

4 green tea bags
2 tablespoons ginger, peeled and sliced

½ cup chopped mint leaves
Juice of 1 lemon or 4 key limes
3 tablespoons honey
Lemon wedges for garnish

Bring 5 cups of spring water to boil, add tea bags, ginger, and mint. Reduce heat to low and steep 5 to 10 minutes, stirring. Pour through strainer into pitcher, add lemon or lime juice and honey. Chill and serve with a lemon wedge.

Variation: Serve hot with ginger, mint, and tea bags remaining as an excellent respiratory soother!

Serves 5 (serving size: 8 fluid ounces)

Servings of fruits and vegetables: none; **diabetes-beating phytonutrients:** catechins

Nutrition information: 50 calories, no protein, no fat, no cholesterol, 14 grams carbohydrate, no dietary fiber, 5 milligrams sodium

❖ *Berry Tart with Cinnamon Oat Crust (Full of Fiber)*

Berry delicious! Berries, with their vessel-protecting anthocyanins, get cozy with cholesterol-reducing oats for a down home dessert.

2 tablespoons canola oil, plus extra to coat pan
⅔ cup old-fashioned oats
1 teaspoon ground cinnamon
½ cup whole-wheat flour
1 tablespoon light brown sugar
¼ teaspoon baking soda

3 tablespoons plain, nonfat yogurt
2 pints mixed berries, such as strawberries, blackberries,
    and blueberries.
¼ cup all-fruit spread
½ teaspoon vanilla extract

Preheat oven to 375°F. Lightly coat a cookie sheet with oil.
Combine oats, cinnamon, flour, sugar, and baking soda in a bowl,
mixing well with a fork. Stir in 2 tablespoons oil and yogurt,
adding more yogurt if dough is too stiff. Pat dough evenly onto
cookie sheet in a 10-inch circle; use a 9-inch pan to make the circle perfect, trimming around the outside with a knife. Pinch the
rim to ¼ inch high; bake 15 minutes to firm and golden. Set aside
to cool and transfer to a serving plate.

Meanwhile, combine berries, fruit spread, and vanilla and
microwave 10 seconds to melt the spread. Spoon the fruit onto
the crust, refrigerate 30 minutes, slice into wedges, and serve.

Serves 4 to 6 (serving size: ⅙ tart)

Servings of fruits and vegetables: 0.5 fruit; **diabetes-beating
phytonutrients:** curcumin, catechin, beta-carotene

Nutrition information: 190 calories, 4 grams protein, 6 grams total fat,
no saturated fat, no cholesterol, 32 grams carbohydrate, 5 grams
dietary fiber, 60 milligrams sodium

Granola

*Oats and nuts deliver a perfect combination of soluble fiber and good
fats.*

3 cups old-fashioned oats (not quick cooking)
1 cup chopped almonds
½ cup chopped walnuts or peanuts (optional)
1 cup sunflower seeds
½ cup flaxseed or soy oil
½ cup honey
1 tablespoon vanilla extract
½ tablespoon cinnamon (freshly ground is best)
¼ teaspoon almond extract (optional)
½ teaspoon sea salt
1 cup dried, organic, unsulfured apricots, chopped
1 cup raisins, currants, or chopped dates

Preheat oven to 325°F. Mix oats, almonds, walnuts or peanuts (if using), and seeds into large bowl. Set aside. Warm up other ingredients, except dried fruit, in a saucepan, and then pour over oat mixture, tossing thoroughly. Spread oat mixture onto cookie sheet or baking pan. Bake for about 20 minutes, stirring granola occasionally, until evenly toasted. Let cool and then toss in a large bowl with dried fruit. Store in an airtight container in a cool, dry place for up to one month.

Makes 7.5 cups (serving size: ¼ cup)

Servings of fruits and vegetables: 0.5 fruit; **diabetes-beating phytonutrients:** glutathione, beta-sitosterol, quercetin, saponins, epicatechin

---

Nutrition information: 180 calories, 4 grams protein, 10 grams total fat, 1 gram saturated fat, no cholesterol, 19 grams carbohydrate, 2 grams dietary fiber, 25 milligrams sodium

---

✣ *Apple and Date Muffins (Full of Fiber)*

Each one of these morsels delivers 5 grams of fiber to keep blood sugar on an even keel.

4 cups apples, peeled, cored, and chopped
½ cup sugar
2 large eggs
¼ cup canola oil
2 teaspoons vanilla extract
2 cups whole-wheat flour
2 teaspoons baking soda
2 teaspoons ground cinnamon
½ teaspoon sea salt
½ cup chopped dates
1 cup chopped walnuts
½ cup unsweetened applesauce
¼ cup fat-free plain yogurt
Canola oil spray

Preheat oven to 350°F. In a large bowl, combine all the ingredients, except for canola oil spray, and mix well. Spray a 12-serving muffin pan with the canola oil and fill each compartment ⅔ full with the apple mixture. Bake for 40 minutes or until golden brown.

Serves 12 (serving size: 1 muffin)

Servings of fruits and vegetables: 0.5 fruit; **diabetes-beating phytonutrients:** beta-sitosterol, phytoestrogens, beta-carotene, beta-stigmasterol

Nutrition information: 270 calories, 6 grams protein, 12 grams total fat, 1.5 grams saturated fat, 35 milligrams cholesterol, 37 grams carbohydrate, 5 grams dietary fiber, 270 milligrams sodium

*A*pricot and Almond Baklava

Baklava is a Middle Eastern specialty, and our recipe gets fruity with carotenoid-rich apricots. Phyllo dough sheets, made without hydrogenated oils, can be found in the frozen section of health-food stores and usually come in twin 8-ounce packages.

¾ cup dried apricots
⅔ cup orange juice
1 large egg
4 ounces nonhydrogenated phyllo dough pastry
Canola oil spray
⅔ cup slivered almonds
⅓ cup honey

Preheat oven to 350°F. Simmer apricots in orange juice until soft, about 10 minutes. Drain and cool. Puree apricots with egg in food processor until smooth. In an 8-inch square baking pan, lay 6 phyllo dough sheets that have been sprayed with canola oil in between the layers. The phyllo sheets should fit the pan perfectly; otherwise trim the edges and discard scraps. Spread half of the almonds on top. Add 3 layers of phyllo sheets, sprayed with canola oil in between the layers. Add the apricot and egg mixture. Top with another 3 layers of phyllo sheets that have been sprayed with canola oil. Finish with the remaining almonds. Score the top phyllo layer into diamonds. Bake for 30 minutes or until golden. Heat the honey in a microwave for 10 to 15 seconds. As soon as the baklava comes hot out of the oven, drizzle hot honey over the top. Let it cool to room temperature and serve.

Serves 6 (serving size: 1 piece)

Servings of fruits and vegetables: 1.25 fruit; **diabetes-beating phytonutrients:** quercetin, phytoestrogens, beta-sitosterol, beta-carotene

Nutrition information: 340 calories, 8 grams protein, 14 grams total fat, 1.5 grams saturated fat, 35 milligrams cholesterol, 48 grams carbohydrate, 4 grams dietary fiber, 105 milligrams sodium

Mango and Cranberry Bread Pudding

A bread pudding rich in antioxidants? Leave it to us! This delicious combination makes liberal use of sugar-balancing spice, plus almonds, cranberries, and mango to boot.

1 cup orange juice
¾ cup chopped dried mango
½ cup dried cranberries
¾ cup chopped fresh mango
1½ cups vanilla soy milk
1 large egg
1 large egg white
2 tablespoons frozen apple juice concentrate
1 pinch nutmeg
1 pinch ground cloves

½ teaspoon ground cinnamon
1 teaspoon vanilla extract
½ whole-grain baguette cut into ⅓-inch-thick slices
Canola oil spray
½ cup slivered almonds, toasted

Preheat oven to 350°F. In a large saucepan, combine orange juice, dried mango, and dried cranberries. Simmer for 5 minutes. Remove from the heat; add fresh mango, and let it sit for 10 minutes. In a large bowl, mix together soy milk, egg, egg white, apple juice concentrate, spices, and vanilla extract. Whisk until well combined. Add bread slices and let it sit for 10 minutes.

In 8-inch pie pan sprayed with canola oil, place one layer of bread slices and top with ⅓ of the mango mixture. Place another layer of bread slices followed by another ⅓ of the mango mix. Add the last layer of bread slices and finish with the last ⅓ of the mango mix. Sprinkle the toasted almonds on top. Cover with aluminum foil. Bake for 30 minutes. Uncover and bake for another 10 minutes. Serve warm.

Serves 6 (serving size: ⅙ bread pudding)

Servings of fruits and vegetables: 1.5 fruits; **diabetes-beating phytonutrients:** phytoestrogens, genistein, quercetin, beta-carotene, beta-sitosterol

Nutrition information: 260 calories, 8 grams protein, 8 grams total fat, 1 gram saturated fat, 35 milligrams cholesterol, 43 grams carbohydrate, 3 grams dietary fiber, 220 milligrams sodium

Appendix
Converting to Metrics

Measurement Conversions

We have included the following tables so you can easily convert measuring ingredients.

Volume Measurement Conversions	
U.S.	**Metric**
¼ teaspoon	1.25 ml
½ teaspoon	2.5 ml
¾ teaspoon	3.75 ml
1 teaspoon	5 ml
1 tablespoon	15 ml
¼ cup	62.5 ml
½ cup	125 ml
¾ cup	187.5 ml
1 cup	250 ml

Weight Conversion Measurements	
U.S.	**Metric**
1 ounce	28.4 g
8 ounces	227.5 g
16 ounces (1 pound)	455 g

Temperature Conversions

We've also included the following table and calculations so you can easily convert cooking temperatures for our recipes.

Cooking Temperature Conversions	
Celsius/Centigrade	0°C and 100°C are arbitrarily placed at the melting and boiling points of water and standard to the metric system
Fahrenheit	Fahrenheit established 0°F as the stabilized temperature when equal amounts of ice, water, and salt are mixed.

To convert temperatures in Fahrenheit to Celsius, use this formula:

$$C = (F - 32) \times 0.5555$$

So, for example, if you are baking at 350°F and want to know that temperature in Celsius, use this calculation:

$$C = (350 - 32) \times 0.5555 = 176.66°C$$

Selected References

Chapter 1: Understanding Diabetes

Centers for Disease Control and Prevention. Centers for Disease Control and Prevention: Diabetes Surveillance Report. Atlanta, GA: U.S. Department of Health and Human Services, 1999.

Grundy, S.M., I. J. Benjamin, G. L. Burke, et al. "Diabetes and Cardiovascular Disease: a Statement for Healthcare Professionals from the American Heart Association." *Circulation* 100 (1999): 1134–46.

Gu, K., C. C. Cowie, and M. I. Harris. "Diabetes and Decline in Heart Disease Mortality in U.S. Adults." *JAMA* 281 (1999): 1291–97.

Haffner, S. M., S. Lehto, T. Ronnemaa, K. Pyorala, M. Laakso. "Mortality from Coronary Heart Disease in Subjects with Type 2 Diabetes and in Nondiabetic Subjects with and Without Prior Myocardial Infarction." *New England Journal of Medicine* 339 (1998): 229–34.

Harris, M. I. "Health Care and Health Status and Outcomes for Patients with Type 2 Diabetes." *Diabetes Care* 23 (2000): 754–58.

Juhan-Vague, I., M. C. Alessi, P. Vague. "Thrombogenic and Fibrinolytic Factors and Cardiovascular Risk in Non-Insulin-Dependent Diabetes Mellitus." *Annals of Medicine* 28 (1996): 371–80.

Miettinen, H., S. Lehto, V. Salomaa, et al. "Impact of Diabetes on Mortality After the First Myocardial Infarction. The FINMONICA Myocardial Infarction Register Study Group." *Diabetes Care* 21 (1998): 69–75.

Roman, S. H., and M. I. Harris. "Management of Diabetes Mellitus from a Public Health Perspective." *Endocrinololgy and Metabolism Clinics of North America* 26 (1997): 443–74.

Wingard, D. L., and E. Barrett-Connor. "Heart Disease and Diabetes." In *Diabetes in America*, ed. National Diabetes Data Group. Washington, DC: National Institutes of Health, NIDDK. NIH publication no. 95-1468,

Chapter 2: Taking Control of Diabetes

Castaneda, C. "Diabetes Control with Physical Activity and Exercise." *Nutritional Clinical Care* 6 (May–Sept. 2003): 89–96.

National Institutes of Health. "Clinical Guidelines on the Identification, Evaluation, and Treatment of Overweight and Obesity in Adults—the Evidence Report." *Obesity Research* 6, supplement 2 (September 1998): 51S–209S.

Chapter 3: The Link: Insulin Resistance, Diabetes, and Metabolic Syndrome

Ajani, U. A., E. S. Ford, and A. H. Mokdad. "Dietary Fiber and C-Reactive Protein: Findings from National Health and Nutrition Examination Survey Data." *Journal of Nutrition* 134 (2004): 1181–85.

Aronson, D., P. Bartha, O. Zinder, A. Kerner, E. Shitman, W. Markiewicz, G. J. Brook, and Y. Levy. "Association Between Fasting Glucose and C-Reactive Protein in Middle-Aged Subjects." *Diabetic Medicine* 21 (2004): 39–44.

Baer, D. J., J. T. Judd, B. A. Clevidence, and R. P. Tracy. "Dietary Fatty Acids Affect Plasma Markers of Inflammation in Healthy Men Fed Controlled Diets: A Randomized Crossover Study." *American Journal of Clinical Nutrition* 79 (2004): 969–73.

Brown, L., B. Rosner, W. C. Willett, and F. M. Sacks. "Cholesterol-Lowering Effects of Dietary Fiber: A Meta-Analysis." *American Journal of Clinical Nutrition* 69 (1999): 30–42.

Ford, E. S., A. H. Mokdad, and S. Liu. "Healthy Eating Index and C-Reactive Protein Concentration: Findings from the National Health and Nutrition Examination Survey III, 1988–1994." *European Journal of Clinical Nutrition* 59 (2005 Feb.): 278–83.

Fung, T. T., F. B. Hu, M. A. Pereira, et al. "Whole-Grain Intake and the Risk of Type 2 Diabetes: A Prospective Study in Men." *American Journal of Clinical Nutrition* 76 (2002): 535–40.

Gao, X., O. I. Bermudez, and K. L. Tucker. "Plasma C-Reactive Protein and Homocysteine Concentrations Are Related to Frequent Fruit and Vegetable Intake in Hispanic and Non-Hispanic White Elders." *Journal of Nutrition* 134 (2004): 913–18.

Grundy, S. "Inflammation, Metabolic Syndrome, and Diet Responsiveness." *Circulation* 108 (2003): 126.

Hou, D. X., M. Fujii, N. Terahara, and M. Yoshimoto. "Molecular Mechanisms Behind the Chemopreventive Effects of Anthocyanidins." *Journal of Biomedicine and Biotechnology* 5 (2004): 321–25.

King, D. E., B. M. Egan, and M. E. Geesey. "Relation of Dietary Fat and Fiber to Elevation of C-Reactive Protein." *American Journal of Cardiology* 92 (Dec. 1, 2003): 1335–39.

Knekt, P., J. Kumpulainen, R. Jarvinen, H. Rissanen, M. Heliovaara, A. Reunanen, T. Hakulinen, and A. Aromaa. "Flavonoid Intake and Risk of Chronic Diseases." *American Journal of Clinical Nutrition* 76 (2002): 560–68.

Lee, Y. H., and R. E. Pratley. "The Evolving Role of Inflammation in Obesity and the Metabolic Syndrome." *Current Diabetes Report* 5 (2005): 70–75.

Lichtenstein, A. H., A. T. Erkkila, B. Lamarche, U. S. Schwab, S. M. Jalbert, and L. M. Ausman. "Influence of Hydrogenated Fat and Butter on CVD Risk Factors: Remnant-Like Particles, Glucose and Insulin, Blood Pressure and C-Reactive Protein." *Atherosclerosis* 171 (Nov. 2003): 97–107.

Liu, S., W. C. Willett, M. J. Stampfer, et al. "A Prospective Study of Dietary Glycemic Load, Carbohydrate Intake, and Risk of Coronary Heart Disease in U.S. Women." *American Journal of Clinical Nutrition* 71 (2000): 1455–61.

Lopez-Garcia, E., M. B. Schulze, T. T. Fung, J. B. Meigs, N. Rifai, J. E. Manson, and F. B. Hu. "Major Dietary Patterns Are Related to Plasma Concentrations of Markers of Inflammation and Endothelial Dysfunction." *American Journal of Clinical Nutrition* 80 (2004): 1029–35.

Maron, D. J. "Flavonoids for Reduction of Atherosclerotic Risk." *Current Atherosclerosis Reports* 6 (Jan. 2004): 73–78.

McKeown, N. M., J. B. Meigs, S. Liu, E. Saltzman, P. W. Wilson, and P. F. Jacques. "Carbohydrate Nutrition, Insulin Resistance, and the Prevalence of the Metabolic Syndrome in the Framingham Offspring Cohort." *Diabetes Care* 27 (2004): 538–46.

Mozaffarian, D., T. Pischon, S. E. Hankinson, N. Rifai, K. Joshipura, W. C. Willett, and E. B. Rimm. "Dietary Intake of Trans Fatty Acids and Systemic Inflammation in Women." *American Journal of Clinical Nutrition* 79 (2004): 606–12.

National Cholesterol Education Program, Third Report of the Expert Panel on Detection, Evaluation, and Treatment of High Blood Cholesterol in Adults (Adult Treatment Panel III), National Heart, Lung, and Blood Institute, National Institutes of Health, May 2001.

National Heart Lung Blood Institute, National Institutes of Health. nhlbi.nih.gov.

National Institutes of Health, Office of Dietary Supplements. dietary-supplements.info.nih.gov/index.aspx.

Pereira, M. A., E. O'Reilly, K. Augustsson, et al. "Dietary Fiber and Risk of Coronary Heart Disease: A Pooled Analysis of Cohort Studies." *Archives of Internal Medicine* 164 (2004): 370–76.

Rimm, E. B., A. Ascherio, E. Giovannucci, D. Spiegelman, M. J. Stampfer, and W. C. Willett. "Vegetable, Fruit, and Cereal Fiber Intake and Risk of Coronary Heart Disease Among Men." *JAMA* 275 (1996): 447–51.

Schulze, M. B., S. Liu, E. B. Rimm, J. E. Manson, W. C. Willett, and F. B. Hu. "Glycemic Index, Glycemic Load, and Dietary Fiber Intake and Incidence of Type 2 Diabetes in Younger and Middle-Aged Women." *American Journal of Clinical Nutrition* 80 (2004): 348–56.

Simin Liu, J., E. Manson, J. E. Buring, M. J. Stampfer, W. C. Willett, and P. M. Ridker. "Relation Between a Diet with a High Glycemic Load and Plasma Concentrations of High-Sensitivity C-Reactive Protein in Middle-Aged Women." *American Journal of Clinical Nutrition* 75 (Mar. 2002): 492–98.

van Herpen-Broekmans, W. M., I. A. Klopping-Ketelaars, M. L. Bots, C. Kluft, H. Princen, H. F. Hendriks, L. B. Tijburg, G. van Poppel, and A. F. Kardinaal. "Serum Carotenoids and Vitamins in Relation to Markers of Endothelial Function and Inflammation." *European Journal of Epidemiology* 19 (2004): 915–21.

van Horn, L. "Fiber, Lipids, and Coronary Heart Disease. A Statement for Healthcare Professionals from the Nutrition Committee, American Heart Association." *Circulation* 95 (1997): 2701–4.

Chapter 4: Fats, Carbs, and Diabetes

Ajani, U. A., E. S. Ford, and A. H. Mokdad. "Dietary Fiber and C-Reactive Protein: Findings from National Health and Nutrition Examination Survey Data." *Journal of Nutrition* 134 (2004): 1181–85.

American Diabetes Association. "Nutritional Recommendations and Principles for Individuals with Diabetes Mellitus." *Diabetes Care* 21 (1998): 532–35

Anderson, J. W., N. J. Gustafson, C. A. Bryant, and J. Tietyen-Clark. "Dietary Fiber and Diabetes: A Comprehensive Review and Practical Application." *Journal of the American Dietetic Association* 87 (1987): 1189–97.

Anderson, J. W., and T. J. Hanna. "Impact of Nondigestible Carbohydrates on Serum Lipoproteins and Risk for Cardiovascular Disease." *Journal of Nutrition* 129 (1999): 1457S–1466S.

Bantle, J. "Clinical Aspects of Sucrose and Fructose Metabolism." *Diabetes Care* 12 (1984): 56–61.

Berry, E. M. "Dietary Fatty Acids in the Management of Diabetes Mellitus." *American Journal of Clinical Nutrition* 66 (1997): 991S–997S.

Bhathena, S. J., and M. T. Velasquez. "Beneficial Role of Dietary Phytoestrogens in Obesity and Diabetes." *American Journal of Clinical Nutrition* 76 (2002): 1191–1201.

Brand, J. C., P. L. Nicholson, A. W. Thorburn, and A. S. Truswell. "Food Processing and the Glycemic Index." *American Journal of Clinical Nutrition* 42 (1985): 1192–96.

Brown, L., B. Rosner, W. C. Willett, and F. M. Sacks. "Cholesterol-Lowering Effects of Dietary Fiber: A Meta-Analysis." *American Journal of Clinical Nutrition* 69 (1999): 30–42.

Fuchs, C. S., E. L. Giovannucci, G. A. Colditz, et al. "Dietary Fiber and the Risk of Colorectal Cancer and Adenoma in Women." *New England Journal of Medicine* 340 (1999): 169–176.

Fung, T. T., F. B. Hu, M. A. Pereira, et al. "Whole-Grain Intake and the Risk of Type 2 Diabetes: A Prospective Study in Men." *American Journal of Clinical Nutrition* 76 (2002): 535–40.

Greenwald, P., E. Lanza, B. Trock, and G. A. Eddy. "Dietary Fiber in the Reduction of Colon Cancer Risk." *Journal of the American Dietetic Association* 87 (1987): 1178–88.

Hallfrisch, J., FACN, and K. M. Behall. "Mechanisms of the Effects of Grains on Insulin and Glucose Responses." *Journal of the American College of Nutrition* 19 (2000): 320S–325S.

"Health Implications of Dietary Fiber—Position of ADA." *Journal of the American Dietetic Association* 97 (1997): 1157–59.

Jalili, T., R. E. C. Wildman, and D. M. Medeiros. "Nutraceutical Roles of Dietary Fiber." *Journal of Nutraceuticals, Functional, and Medical Foods* 2 (2000): 19–34.

Jenkins, D. J., C. W. Kendall, L. S. Augustin, et al. "Glycemic Index: Overview of Implications in Health and Disease." *American Journal of Clinical Nutrition* 76 (2002): 266S–273S.

Khor, G. L. "Dietary Fat Quality: A Nutritional Epidemiologist's View." *Asia Pacific Journal of Clinical Nutrition* 13 (Aug. 2004)): S22.

Liese, A. D., M. Schulz, C. G. Moore, and E. J. Mayer-Davis. "Dietary Patterns, Insulin Sensitivity and Adiposity in the Multi-Ethnic Insulin Resistance Atherosclerosis Study Population." *British Journal of Nutrition* 92 (Dec. 2004): 973–84.

Liu, S. "Insulin Resistance, Hyperglycemia and Risk of Major Chronic Diseases—a Dietary Perspective." *Proceedings of the Nutrition Society of Australia* 22 (1998): 140–50.

Liu, S. "Intake of Refined Carbohydrates and Whole Grain Foods in Relation to Risk of Type 2 Diabetes Mellitus and Coronary Heart Disease." *American Journal of Clinical Nutrition* 21 (2002): 298–306.

Liu, S., W. C. Willett, J. E. Manson, F. B. Hu, B. Rosner, and G. Colditz. "Relation Between Changes in Intakes of Dietary Fiber and Grain Products and Changes in Weight and Development of Obesity Among Middle-Aged Women." *American Journal of Clinical Nutrition* 78 (Nov. 2003): 920–27.

Liu, S., W. C. Willett, M. J. Stampfer, et al. "A Prospective Study of Dietary Glycemic Load, Carbohydrate Intake and Risk of Coronary Heart Disease in U.S. Women." *American Journal of Clinical Nutrition* 71 (2000): 1455–61.

Louheranta, A. M., E. S. Sarkkinen, H. M. Vidgren, U. S. Schwab, and M. I. Uusitupa. "Association of the Fatty Acid Profile of Serum Lipids with Glucose and Insulin Metabolism During 2 Fat-Modified Diets in Subjects with Impaired Glucose Tolerance." *American Journal of Clinical Nutrition* 76 (Aug. 2002): 331–37.

Ludwig, D. S. "Diet and Development of Insulin Resistance Syndrome." *Asia Pacific Journal of Clinical Nutrition* 12 (2003): S4.

Ludwig, D. "Dietary Glycemic Index and Obesity." *Journal of Nutrition* 130 (2000): 280S–283S.

Manco, M., M. Calvani, and G. Mingrove. "Effects of Dietary Fatty Acids on Insulin Sensitivity and Secretion." *Diabetes, Obesity, and Metabolism* 6 (Nov. 2004): 402–13.

Marlett, J. A. "Content and Composition of Dietary Fiber in 117 Frequently Consumed Foods." *Journal of the American Dietetic Association* 92 (1992): 175–86.

Marlett, J. A., M. I. McBurney, J. L. Slavin, and American Dietetic Association. "Position of the American Dietetic Association: Health Implications of Dietary Fiber." *American Journal of Clinical Nutrition* 102 (2002): 993–1000.

McKeown, N. M., J. B. Meigs, S. Liu, E. Saltzman, P. W. Wilson, and P. F. Jacques. "Carbohydrate Nutrition, Insulin Resistance, and the Prevalence of the Metabolic Syndrome in the Framingham Offspring Cohort." *Diabetes Care* 27 (2004): 538–46.

McKeown, N. M., J. B. Meigs, S. Liu, P. W. Wilson, P. F. Jacques. "Whole-Grain Intake Is Favorably Associated with Metabolic Risk Factors for Type 2 Diabetes and Cardiovascular Disease in the Framingham Offspring Study." *American Journal of Clinical Nutrition* 76 (Aug. 2002): 390–98.

Meyer, K. A., L. H. Kushi, D. R. Jacobs, Jr., J. Slavin, T. A. Sellers, and A. R. Folsom. "Carbohydrates, Dietary Fiber, and Incident Type 2 Diabetes in Older Women." *American Journal of Clinical Nutrition* 71 (2000): 921–30.

Mozaffarian, D., T. Pischon, S. E. Hankinson, N. Rifai, K. Joshipura, W. C. Willett, E. B. Rimm. "Dietary Intake of Trans Fatty Acids and Systemic Inflammation in Women." *American Journal of Clinical Nutrition* 79 (Apr. 2004): 606–12.

National Institutes of Health. NIH Consensus Development Conference Statement on Diet and Exercise, Bethesda, MD, U.S. Department of Health and Human Services, 1986.

Nobukata, H., T. Ishikawa, M. Obata, and Y. Shibutani. "Long-Term Administration of Highly Purified Eicosapentaenoic Acid Ethyl Ester Prevents Diabetes and Abnormalities of Blood Coagulation in Male WBN/Kob Rats." *Metabolism* 49 (July 2000): 912–19.

Okuda, Y., M. Mizutani, M. Ogawa, H. Sone, M. Asano, Y. Asakura, M. Isaka, S. Suzuki, Y. Kawakami, J. B. Field, and K. Yamashita. "Long-Term Effects of Eicosapentaenoic Acid on Diabetic Peripheral Neuropathy and Serum Lipids in Patients with Type II Diabetes Mellitus." *Journal of Diabetes and Its Complications* 10 (Sept.–Oct. 1996): 280–87.

Omega-3 Sources, USDA. nal.usda.gov.

Pereira, M. A., E. O'Reilly, K. Augustsson, et al. "Dietary Fiber and Risk of Coronary Heart Disease: A Pooled Analysis of Cohort Studies." *Archives of Internal Medicine* 164 (2004): 370–76.

Popov, D., M. Simionescu, and P. R. Shepherd. "Saturated Fat Induces Moderate Diabetes and Severe Glumerulosclerosis in Hampsters." *Diabetologica* 46 (Oct. 2003): 1408–18.

Questions and Answers on Trans Fat Proposed Rule. U.S. Food and Drug Administration. Center for Food Safety and Applied Nutrition. November 1999. cfsan.fds.gov.

Rimm, E. B., A. Ascherio, E. Giovannucci, D. Spiegelman, M. J. Stampfer, and W. C. Willett. "Vegetable, Fruit, and Cereal Fiber Intake and Risk of Coronary Heart Disease Among Men." *JAMA* 275 (1996): 447–51.

Rustan, A. C., M. S. Nenseter, and C. A. Drevon. "Omega-3 and Omega-6 Fatty Acids in the Insulin Resistance Syndrome. Lipid and Lipoprotein Metabolism and Atherosclerosis." *Annals of the New York Academy of Sciences* 827 (September 20, 1997): 310–26.

Scheppach, W., S. Bingham, M. C. Boutron-Ruault, et al. "WHO Consensus Statement on the Role of Nutrition in Colorectal Cancer." *European Journal of Cancer Prevention* 8 (1999): 57–62.

Schulze, M. B., S. Liu, E. B. Rimm, J. E. Manson, W. C. Willett, and F. B. Hu. "Glycemic Index, Glycemic Load, and Dietary Fiber Intake and Incidence of Type 2 Diabetes in Younger and Middle-Aged Women." *American Journal of Clinical Nutrition* 80 (2004): 348–56.

Shi, J., K. Arunasalam, D. Yeung, Y. Kakuda, G. Mittal, and Y. Jiang. "Saponins from Edible Legumes: Chemistry, Processing, and Health Benefits." *Journal of Medicinal Food* 7 (Spring 2004): 67–78.

Simopoulos, A. P. "Essential Fatty Acids in Health and Chronic Disease." *American Journal of Clinical Nutrition* 70 (Sept. 1999): 560S–569S.

Song, Y., J. E. Manson, J. E. Buring, S. Liu. "A Prospective Study of Red Meat Consumption and Type 2 Diabetes in Middle-Aged and Elderly Women: The Women's Health Study." *Diabetes Care* 27 (Sept. 2004): 2108–15.

Stark, A. H., and Z. Madar. "Olive Oil as a Functional Food: Epidemiology and Nutritional Approaches." *Nutrition Reviews* 60 (June 2002): 170–76.

Tanasescu, M., E. Cho, J. E. Manson, and F. B. Hu. "Dietary Fat and Cholesterol and the Risk of Cardiovascular Disease Among Women with Type 2 Diabetes." *American Journal of Clinical Nutrition* 79 (June 2004): 999–1005.

Thompson, L. U., J. H. Yoon, D. J. Jenkins, T. M. Wolever, and A. L. Jenkins. "Relationship Between Polyphenol Intake and Blood Glucose Response of Normal and Diabetic Individuals." *American Journal of Clinical Nutrition* 139 (1984): 745–51.

Thorne, M. J., L. U. Thompson, and D. J. Jenkins. "Factors Affecting Starch Digestibility and the Glycemic Response with Special Reference to Legumes." *American Journal of Clinical Nutrition* 38 (1983): 481–88.

Todd, P. A., P. Benfield, and K. L. Goa. "Guar Gum: A Review of its Pharmacological Properties, and Use as a Dietary Adjunct in Hypercholesterolaemia." *Drugs* 39 (1990): 917–28.

Todd, S., M. Woodward, H. Tunstall-Pedoe, and C. Bolton-Smith. "Dietary Antioxidant Vitamins and Fiber in the Etiology of Cardiovascular Disease and All-Causes Mortality: Results from the Scottish Heart Health Study." *American Journal of Epidemiology* 150 (1999): 1073–80.

Van Dam, R. M., W. C. Willett, E. B. Rimm, M. J. Stampfer, and F. B. Hu. "Dietary Fat and Meat Intake in Relation to Risk of Type 2 Diabetes in Men." *Diabetes Care* 25 (Mar. 2002): 417–24.

Van Horn, L. "Fiber, Lipids, and Coronary Heart Disease. A Statement for Healthcare Professionals from the Nutrition Committee, American Heart Association." *Circulation* 95 (1997): 2701–4.

Veldman, F. J., C. H. Nair, H. H. Vorster, et al. "Dietary Pectin Influences Fibrin Network Structure in Hypercholesterolaemic Subjects." *Thrombosis Research* 86 (1997): 183–96.

"What You Need to Know About Mercury in Fish and Shellfish." 2004 EPA and FDA advice, cfsan.fda.gov/~dms/admehg3.

Wolever, T., and C. Bolognesi. "Prediction of Glucose and Insulin Responses of Normal Subjects After Consuming Mixed Meals Varying in Energy, Protein, Fat, Carbohydrate and Glycemic Index." *Nutrition* 1126 (1992): 2807–12.

Wolever, T. M., D. J. Jenkins, A. L. Jenkins, and R. G. Josse. "The Glycemic Index: Methodology and Clinical Implications." *American Journal of Clinical Nutrition* 54 (1991): 846–54.

Wolk, A., J. E. Manson, M. J. Stampfer, et al. "Long-Term Intake of Dietary Fiber and Decreased Risk of Coronary Heart Disease Among Women." *JAMA* 281 (1999): 1998–2004.

Yoon, J. H., L. U. Thompson, and D. J. Jenkins. "The Effect of Phytic Acid on in Vitro Rate of Starch Digestibility and Blood Glucose Response." *American Journal of Clinical Nutrition* 38 (1983): 835–42.

Ziegler, R. G. "Vegetables, Fruits, and Carotenoids and the Risk of Cancer." *American Journal of Clinical Nutrition* 53 (1991): 251S–259S.

Chapter 5: Antioxidants, Phytonutrients, and Other Diabetes-Fighting Nutrients

Ames, B. N. and L. S. Gold. "Endogenous Mutagens and the Causes of Aging and Cancer." *Mutation Research* 250 (1991): 3–16.

Andersson, T. L., J. Matz, G. A. Ferns, and E. E. Anggard. "Vitamin E Reverses Cholesterol-Induced Endothelial Dysfunction in the Rabbit Coronary Circulation." *Atherosclerosis* 111 (1994): 39–45.

Avena, R., S. Arora, B. J. Carmody, K. Cosby, and A. N. Sidawy. "Thiamine (Vitamin B_1) Protects Against Glucose- and Insulin-Mediated

Proliferation of Human Infragenicular Arterial Smooth Muscle Cells." *Annals of Vascular Surgery* 14 (Jan. 2000): 37–43.

Babu, P. S., and K. Srinivasan. "Influence of Dietary Curcumin and Cholesterol on the Progression of Experimentally Induced Diabetes in Albino Rat." *Molecular and Cellular Biochemistry* 152 (1995): 13–21.

Barbagallo, M., L. J. Dominguez, M. R. Tagliamonte, L. M. Resnick, and G. Paolisso. "Effects of Vitamin E and Glutathione on Glucose Metabolism: Role of Magnesium." *Hypertension* 34 (Oct. 1999): 1002–6.

Beatty, S., H. Koh, M. Phil, D. Henson, and M. Boulton. "The Role of Oxidative Stress in the Pathogenesis of Age-Related Macular Degeneration." *Survey of Ophthalmology* 45 (Sept.–Oct. 2000): 115–34.

Berr, C., B. Balansard, J. Arnaud, A. M. Roussel, A. Alperovitch. "Cognitive Decline Is Associated with Systemic Oxidative Stress: The EVA Study. Etude du Vieillissement Arteriel." *Journal of the American Geriatric Society* 48 (Oct. 2000): 1285–91.

Bhathena, S. J., and M. T. Velasquez. "Beneficial Role of Dietary Phytoestrogens in Obesity and Diabetes." *American Journal of Clinical Nutrition* 76 (Dec. 2002): 1191–1201.

Bordia, A., S. K. Verma, and K. C. Srivastava. "Effect of Garlic (Allium Sativum) on Blood Lipids, Blood Sugar, Fibrinogen and Fibrinolytic Activity in Patients with Coronary Artery Disease." *Prostaglandins, Leukotrienes, and Essential Fatty Acids* 58 (Apr. 1998): 257–63.

Brown, L., E. B. Rimm, J. M. Seddon, E. L. Giovannucci, L. Chasan-Taber, D. Spiegelman, W. C. Willett, and S. E. Hankinson. "A Prospective Study of Carotenoid Intake and Risk of Cataract Extraction in U.S. Men." *American Journal of Clinical Nutrition* 170 (Oct. 1999): 517–24.

Centers for Disease Control and Prevention. Centers for Disease Control and Prevention: Diabetes Surveillance Report. Atlanta, GA: U.S. Department of Health and Human Services, 1999.

Cohen-Boulakia, F., P. E. Valensi, H. Boulahdour, R. Lestrade, J. F. Dufour-Lamartinie, C. Hort-Legrand, and A. Behar. "In Vivo Sequential Study of Skeletal Muscle Capillary Permeability in Diabetic Rats: Effect of Anthocyanosides." *Metabolism* 49 (July 2000): 880–85.

Cowell, R. C., and J. W. Russell. "Nirosaative Injury and Antioxidant Therapy in the Management of Diabetic Neuropathy." *Journal of Investigative Medicine* 52 (2004): 33–44.

Dashwood, R. H. "Indol-3-Carbinolanticarcinogen or Tumor Promoter in Brassica Vegetables." *Chemico-Biological Interactions* 110 (1998): 1–5.

Davi, G., G. Ciabattoni, A. Consoli, et al. "In Vivo Formation of 8-Iso-Prostaglandin F2a and Platelet Activation in Diabetes Mellitus. Effects of Improved Metabolic Control and Vitamin E Supplementation." *Circulation* 99 (1999): 224–29.

Diaz-Arrastia, R. "Homocysteine and Neurologic Disease." *Archives of Neurology* 57 (Oct. 2000): 1422–27.

Dickinson, P. J., A. L. Carrington, G. S. Frost, and A. J. Boulton. "Neurovascular Disease, Antioxidants and Glycation in Diabetes." *Diabetes/Metabolism Research and Reviews* 18 (July–Aug. 2002): 260–72.

Exner, M., M. Hermann, R. Hofbauer, et al. "Genistein Prevents the Glucose Autooxidation Mediated Atherogenic Modification of Low Density Lipoprotein." *Free Radical Research* 34 (Jan. 2001): 101–12.

Freund, H., S. Atamian, and J. E. Fischer. "Chromium Deficiency During Total Parenteral Nutrition." *JAMA* 241 (1979): 496–98.

Grundy, S. M., I. J. Benjamin, G. L. Burke, et al. "Diabetes and Cardiovascular Disease: A Statement for Healthcare Professionals from the American Heart Association." *Circulation* 100 (1999): 1134–46.

Guan, X., J. J. Matte, P. K. Ku, et al. "High Chromium Yeast Supplementation Improves Glucose Tolerance in Pigs by Decreasing Hepatic Extraction of Insulin." *Journal of Nutrition* 130 (2000): 1274–79.

Haffner, S. M., S. Lehto, T. Ronnemaa, K. Pyorala, and M. Laakso. "Mortality from Coronary Heart Disease in Subjects with Type 2 Diabetes and in Nondiabetic Subjects with and Without Prior Myocardial Infarction." *New England Journal of Medicine* 339 (1998): 229–34.

Harvard School of Public Health, Division of Cancer Prevention (website): Taking Antioxidants for Cancer Prevention: A Leap of Faith. hsph.harvard.edu/cancer/publications/source/v9n1/focus.

Haskins, K., J. Kench, K. Powers, B. Bradley, S. Pugazhenthi, and J. Reusch. "Role for Oxidative Stress in the Regeneration of Islet Beta Cells?" *Journal of Medical Investigation* 52 (2004): 45–49.

Heber, D., and S. Bowerman. "Applying Science to Changing Dietary Patterns." *Journal of Nutrition* 131 (Nov. 2001): 3078S–3081S.

Heber, D. "Vegetables, Fruits and Phytoestrogens in the Prevention of Diseases." *Journal of Postgraduate Medicine* 50 (Apr.–June 2004): 145–49.

Ho, E., and T. M. Bray. "Antioxidants, NFkappaB Activation, and Diabetogenesis." *Proceedings of the Society for Experimental Biology and Medicine* 222 (1999): 205–13.

Huang, C. N., J. S. Horng, and M. C. Yin. "Antioxidative and Antiglycative Effects of Six Organosulfur Compounds in Low-Density Lipoprotein and Plasma." *Journal of Agricultural and Food Chemistry* 52 (June 2004): 3674–78.

Jacques, P., L. L. T. Chylack Jr., S. E. Hankinson, et al. "Long-Term Nutrient Intake and Early Age-Related Nuclear Lens Opacities." *Archives of Ophthalmology* 119 (2001): 1009–19.

Kaneto, H., Y. Kajimoto, Y. Fujitani, et al. "Oxidative Stress Induces p21 Expression in Pancreatic Islet Cells: Possible Implication in Beta-Cell Dysfunction." *Diabetologia* 42 (1999): 1093–97.

Khamaisi, M., O. Kavel, M. Rosenstock, M. Porat, M. Yuli, N. Kaiser, and A. Rudich. "Effect of Inhibition of Glutathione Synthesis on Insulin Action: In Vivo and in Vitro Studies Using Buthioninesulfoximine." *Biochemical Journal* 349 (July 2000): 579–86.

Knekt, P., J. Kumpulainen, R. Jarvinen, H. Rissanen, M. Heliovaara, A. Reunanen, T. Hakulinen, and A. Aromaa. "Flavonoid Intake and Risk of Chronic Diseases." *American Journal of Clinical Nutrition* 76 (Sept. 2002): 560–68.

Lampeter, E. F., A. Klinghammer, W. A. Scherbaum, et al. "The Deutsche Nicotinamide Intervention Study: An Attempt to Prevent Type 1 Diabetes." *Diabetes* 47 (1998): 980–84.

Liu, R. "Potential Synergy of Phytochemicals in Cancer Prevention: Mechanism of Action." *Journal of Nutrition* 134 (Dec. 2004): 3479S–3485S.

Liu, R. H. "Health Benefits of Fruits and Vegetables Are from Additive and Synergistic Combination of Phytochemicals." *American Journal of Clinical Nutrition* 78 (2003): 517S–520S.

Liu, S. "Insulin Resistance, Hyperglycemia and Risk of Major Chronic Diseases—A Dietary Perspective." Proceedings of the Nutrition Society of Australia 22 (1998): 140–50.

Liu, S., W. C. Willett, M. J. Stampfer, et al. "A Prospective Study of Dietary Glycemic Load, Carbohydrate Intake and Risk of Coronary Heart Disease in U.S. Women." *American Journal of Clinical Nutrition* 71 (2000): 1455–61.

McDermott, J. H. "Antioxidant Nutrients: Current Dietary Recommendations and Research Update." *Journal of the American Pharmaceutical Association* 40 (Nov.–Dec. 2000): 785–99.

Mezei, O., W. J. Banz, R. W. Steger, et al. "Soy Isoflavones Exert Antidiabetic and Hypolipidemic Effects Through PPAR Pathways in Obese Zucker Rats and Murine RAW 264.7 Cells." *Journal of Nutrition* 133 (May 2003): 1238–43.

Michnovicz, J. J., and H. L. Bradlow. 1991. "Altered Estrogen Metabolism and Excretion in Humans Following Consumption of Indole Carbinol." *Nutrition and Cancer* 16 (1991): 59–66.

Montonen, J., P. Knekt, R. Jarvinen, and A. Reunanen. "Dietary Antioxidant Intake and Risk of Type 2 Diabetes." *Diabetes Care* 27 (Feb. 2004): 362–66.

National Institute on Aging Age Page: Life Extension: Science Fact or Science Fiction? U.S. Department of Health and Human Services, Public Health Service, National Institutes of Health, niapublications .org/engagepages/lifeext.asp.

NCI, 5-A-Day Website, Glossary of Phytochemicals. 5aday.gov.

NIA Research Goal B: Understand Healthy Aging Processes Subgoal 1: Unlock The Secrets of Aging, Health, and Longevity, nia.nih.gov/ aboutnia/strategicplan/researchgoalb/subgoal1.

Ou, C. C., S. M. Tsao, M. C. Lin, and M. C. Yin. "Protective Action on Human LDL Against Oxidation and Glycation by Four Organosulfur Compounds Derived from Garlic." *Lipids* 38 (Mar. 2003): 219–24.

Paolisso, G., M. Barbagallo. "Hypertension, Diabetes Mellitus, and Insulin Resistance: The Role of Intracellular Magnesium." *Journal of Hypertension* 10 (1997): 346–55.

Pennathur, S., J. D. Wagner, C. Leeuwenburgh, K. N. Litwak, and J. W. Heinecke. "A Hydroxyl Radical-Like Species Oxidizes Cynomolgus Monkey Artery Wall Proteins in Early Diabetic Vascular Disease." *Journal of Clinical Investigation* 107 (2001): 853–60.

Rasik, A. M., and A. Shukla. "Antioxidant Status in Delayed Healing Type of Wounds." *International Journal of Experimental Pathology* 81 (Aug. 2000): 257–63.

Robertson, P. "Chronic Oxidative Stress as a Mechanism for Glucose Toxicity in Pancreatic Islet Beta Cells in Diabetes." *Journal of Biological Chemistry* 279 (2004): 42351–54.

Romero-Navarro, G., G. Cabrera-Valladares, M. S. German, et al. "Biotin Regulation of Pancreatic Glucokinase and Insulin in Primary Cultured Rat Islets and in Biotin-Deficient Rats." *Endocrinology* 140 (1999): 4595–4600.

Sekiya, K., A. Ohtani, and S. Kusano. "Enhancement of Insulin Sensitivity in Adipocytes by Ginger." *Biofactors.* 22 (2004): 153–56.

Sidhu, G. S., H. Mani, J. P. Gaddipati, A. K. Singh, P. Seth, K. K. Banaudha, G. K. Patnaik, and R. K. Maheshwari. "Curcumin

Enhances Wound Healing in Streptozotocin Induced Diabetic Rats and Genetically Diabetic Mice." *Wound Repair and Regeneration* 7 (Sept.–Oct. 1999): 362–74.

Smith, T. J. "Mechanisms of Carcinogenesis Inhibition by Isothiocyanates." *Expert Opinion on Investigational Drugs* 10 (Dec. 2001): 2167–74.

Tijburg, L. B. M., T. Mattern, J. D. Folts, U. M. Weisgerber, and M. B. Katan. "Tea Flavonoids and Cardiovascular Diseases: A Review." *Critical Reviews in Food Science and Nutrition* 37 (1997): 771–85.

Ting, H. H., F. K. Timimi, K. S. Boles, S. J. Creager, P. Ganz, and M. A. Creager. "Vitamin C Improves Endothelium-Dependent Vasodilation in Patients with Non-Insulin-Dependent Diabetes Mellitus." *Journal of Clinical Investigation* 97 (1996): 22–28.

Tsuda, T., F. Horio, K. Uchida, H. Aoki, and T. Osawa. "Dietary Cyanidin 3-O-beta-D-Glucoside-Rich Purple Corn Color Prevents Obesity and Ameliorates Hyperglycemia in Mice." *Journal of Nutrition* 133 (July 2003): 2125–30.

Tsuda, T., Y. Ueno, H. Aoki, T. Koda, F. Horio, N. Takahashi, T. Kawada, and T. Osawa. "Anthocyanin Enhances Adipocytokine Secretion and Adipocyte-Specific Gene Expression in Isolated Rat Adipocytes." *Biochemical and Biophysical Research Communications* 316 (Mar. 2004): 149–57.

United States Department of Agriculture, Agricultural Research Service. Food and Nutrient Intakes by Individuals in the United States, by Sex and Age, 1994–1996. Nationwide Food Surveys Report No. 96–2, 1998, USDA Washington, DC.

Vaskonen, T. "Dietary Minerals and Modification of Cardiovascular Risk Factors." *Journal of Nutritional Biochemistry* 14 (Sept. 2003): 492–506.

Vincent, A. M., J. W. Russell, P. Low, and E. L. Feldman. "Oxidative Stress in the Pathogenesis of Diabetic Neuropathy." *Endocrine Reviews* 25 (Aug. 2004): 612–28.

Wahlberg, G., L. A. Carlson, J. Wasserman, et al. "Protective Effect of Nicotinamide Against Nephropathy in Diabetic Rats." *Diabetes Research* 2 (1985): 307.

World Cancer Research Fund & American Institute for Cancer Research. *Food, Nutrition, and the Prevention of Cancer: A Global Perspective.* Washington, DC: American Institute for Cancer Research, 1997.

Yeh, Y. Y., and L. Liu. "Cholesterol-Lowering Effect of Garlic Extracts and Organosulfur Compounds: Human and Animal Studies." *Journal of Nutrition* 131 (Mar. 2001): 989S–93S.

Zhang, H., K. Osada, H. Sone, et al. "Biotin Administration Improves the Impaired Glucose Tolerance of Streptozotocin-Induced Diabetic Wistar Rats." *Journal of Nutritional Science and Vitaminology* 43 (1997): 2271–80.

Chapter 6: Diabetes-Beating Foods

Adom, K. K., and R. H. Liu. "Antioxidant Activity of Grains." *Journal of Agricultural and Food Chemistry* 50 (2002): 6182–87.

Adom, K. K., M. E. Sorrells, and R. H. Liu. "Phytochemicals and Antioxidant Activity of Wheat Varieties." *Journal of Agricultural and Food Chemistry* 51 (2003): 7825–34.

Blot, W. J., J. Y. Li, P. R. Taylor, W. Guo, S. Dawsey, G. Q. Wang, C. S. Yang, S. F. Zheng, M. Gail, et al. "Nutrition Intervention Trials in Linxian, China: Supplementation with Specific Vitamin/Mineral Combinations, Cancer Incidence, and Disease-Specific Mortality in the General Population." *Journal of the National Cancer Institute* 85 (1993): 1483–92.

Eberhardt, M. V., C. Y. Lee, and R. H. Liu. "Antioxidant Activity of Fresh Apples." *Nature* 405 (2000): 903–4.

Heber D. "Vegetables, Fruits and Phytoestrogens in the Prevention of Diseases." *Journal of Postgraduate Medicine* 50 (2004): 145–49.

Hennekens, C. H., J. E. Buring, J. E. Manson, M. Stampfer, and B. Rosner. "Lack of Effect of Long-Term Supplementation with ß-Carotene on the Incidence of Malignant Neoplasms and Cardiovascular Disease." *New England Journal of Medicine* 334 (1996): 1145–49.

Jacobs, D., and L. Steffen. "Nutrients, Foods and Dietary Patterns as Exposures in Research: A Framework for Food Synergy." *American Journal of Clinical Nutrition* 78 (Sept. 2003): 508S–513S.

Ommen, G. S., G. E. Goodman, M. D. Thomquist, J. Barnes, and M. R. Cullen. (1996) "Effects of a Combination of ß-Carotene and Vitamin A on Lung Cancer and Cardiovascular Disease." *New England Journal of Medicine* 334 (1996): 1150–55.

Salonen, J. T., K. Nyyssonen, R. Salonen, H. M. Lakka, J. Kaikkonen, E. Porkkala-Sarataho, S. Voutilainen, T. A. Lakka, T. Rissanen, et al. (2000) "Antioxidant Supplementation in Artherosclerosis Prevention (ASAP) Study: A Randomized Trial of the Effect of Vitamins E and C on 3-Year Progression of Carotid Atherosclerosis." *Journal of Internal Medicine* 248 (2000): 377–86.

Slavin, J. "Why Whole Grains Are Protective: Biological Mechanisms." *Proceedings of the Nutrition Society* 62 (Feb. 2003): 129–34.

Stephens, N. G., A. Parsons, P. M. Schofield, F. Kelly, K. Cheeseman, and M. J. Mitchinson. "Randomized Controlled Trial of Vitamin E in Patients with Coronary Disease: Cambridge Heart Antioxidant Study (CHAOS)." *Lancet* 347 (1996): 781–86.

The Alpha-Tocopherol, Beta Carotene Cancer Prevention Study Group. "The Effect of Vitamin E and ß-Carotene on the Incidence of Lung Cancer and Other Cancers in Male Smokers." *New England Journal of Medicine* 330 (1994): 1029–35.

Yusuf, S., G. Dagenais, J. Pogue, J. Bosch, and P. Sleight. (2000) "Vitamin E Supplementation and Cardiovascular Events in High-Risk Patients. The Heart Outcomes Prevention Evaluation Study Investigators." *New England Journal of Medicine* 342 (2000): 154–60.

Chapter 7: Healing Herbs and Spices

Aggarwal, B. B, and S. Shishodia. "Suppression of the Nuclear Factor-κB Activation Pathway by Spice-Derived Phytochemicals: Reasoning for Seasoning." *Annals of the New York Academy of Sciences* 1030 (Dec. 2004): 434–41.

Agrawal P., V. Rai, and R. B. Singh. "Randomized Placebo-Controlled, Single Blind Trial of Holy Basil Leaves in Patients with Noninsulin-Dependent Diabetes Mellitus." *International Journal of Clinical Pharmacology and Therapeutics* 34 (Sept. 1996): 406–9.

Aguiyi, J. C., C. I. Obi, S. S. Gang, and A. C. Igweh. "Hypoglycaemic Activity of Ocimum Gratissimum in Rats." *Fitoterapia* 71 (Aug. 2000): 444–46.

Ali, B. H., and G. Blunden. "Pharmacological and Toxicological Properties of Nigella Sativa." *Phytotherapy Research* 17 (Apr. 2003): 299–305.

al-Sereiti, M. R., K. M. Abu-Amer, and P. Sen. "Pharmacology of Rosemary (Rosmarinus Officinalis Linn.) and Its Therapeutic Potentials." *Indian Journal of Experimental Biology* 37 (Feb. 1999): 124–30.

American Spice Trade Association. astaspice.org.

Anderson, R. A., C. L. Broadhurst, M. M. Polansky, W. F. Schmidt, A. Khan, V. P. Flanagan, N. W. Schoene, and D. J. Graves. "Isolation and Characterization of Polyphenol Type-A Polymers from Cinnamon with Insulin-Like Biological Activity." *Journal of Agricultural and Food Chemistry* 52 (Jan. 14, 2004): 65–70.

Arcila-Lozano, C. C., G. Loarca-Pina, S. Lecona-Uribe, and E. Gonzalez de Mejia. "Oregano: Properties, Composition and Biological Activity." *Archives of Latinoamerican Nutrition* 54 (Mar. 2004): 100–111.

Arun, N., and N. Nalini. "Efficacy of Turmeric on Blood Sugar and Polyol Pathway in Diabetic Albino Rats." *Plant Foods for Human Nutrition* 57 (Winter 2002): 41–52.

Babu, P., and K. Srinivasan. "Amelioration of Renal Lesions Associated with Diabetes by Dietary Curcumin in Streptozotocin Diabetic rats." *Molecular and Cellular Biochemistry* 181 (Apr. 1998): 87–96.

Bordia, A., S. K. Verma, and K. C. Srivastava. "Effect of Ginger (Zingiber Officinale Rosc.) and Fenugreek (Trigonella Foenumgraecum L.) on Blood Lipids, Blood Sugar and Platelet Aggregation in Patients with Coronary Artery Disease." *Prostaglandins, Leukotrienes, and Essential Fatty Acids* 56 (May 1997): 379–84.

Broadhurst, C. L., M. M. Polansky, and R. A. Anderson. "Insulin-Like Biological Activity of Culinary and Medicinal Plant Aqueous Extracts in Vitro." *Journal of Agricultural and Food Chemistry* 48 (Mar. 2000): 849–52.

Choi, E. M., and J. K. Hwang. "Antiinflammatory, Analgesic and Antioxidant Activities of the Fruit of Foeniculum Vulgare." *Fitoterapia* 75 (Sept. 2004): 557–65.

Cook, N. C., and S. Samman. "Flavonoids—Chemistry, Metabolism, Cardioprotective Effects, and Dietary Sources." *Journal of Nutritional Biochemistry* 7 (1996): 66–76.

Dhandapani, S., V. R. Subramanian, S. Rajagopal, and N. Namasivayam. "Hypolipidemic Effect of Cuminum Cyminum L. on Alloxan-Induced Diabetic Rats." *Pharmacology Research* 46 (Sept. 2002): 251–55.

Elson, C. E. "Suppression of Mevalonate Pathway Activities by Dietary Isoprenoids: Protective Roles in Cancer and Cardiovascular Disease." *Journal of Nutrition* 125 (1995): 1666S–72S.

Fuhrman, B., M. Rosenblat, T. Hayek, R. Coleman, M. Aviram. "Ginger Extract Consumption Reduces Plasma Cholesterol, Inhibits LDL Oxidation and Attenuates Development of Atherosclerosis in Atherosclerotic, Apolipoprotein E-Deficient Mice." *Journal of Nutrition* 130 (May 2000): 1124–31.

Guh, J. H., F. N. Ko, T. T. Jong, and C. M. Teng. "Antiplatelet Effect of Gingerol Isolated from Zingiber Officinale." *Journal of Pharmacy and Pharmacology* 47 (Apr. 1995): 329–32.

Khan, A., M. Safdar, M. M. Ali Khan, K. N. Khattak, and R. A. Anderson. "Cinnamon Improves Glucose and Lipids of People with Type 2 Diabetes." *Diabetes Care* 26: (Dec. 2003): 3215–18.

Lal, A. A., T. Kumar, P. B. Murthy, and K. S. Pillai. "Hypolipidemic Effect of Coriandrum Aativum L. in Triton-Induced Hyperlipidemic Rats." *Indian Journal of Experimental Biology* 42 (Sept. 2004): 909–12.

Lemhadri, A., N. A. Zeggwagh, M. Maghrani, H. Jouad, and M. Eddouks. "Anti-Hyperglycaemic Activity of the Aqueous Extract of Origanum Vulgare Growing Wild in Tafilalet Region." *Journal of Ethnopharmacology* 92 (June 2004): 251–56.

Manach, C., F. Regerat, O. Texier, et al. "Bioavailability, Metabolism and Physiological Impact of 4-Oxo-Flavonoids." *Nutrition Research* 16 (1996): 517–44.

McCarty, M. F. "Nutraceutical Resources for Diabetes Prevention— An Update." *Medical Hypotheses* 64 (2005): 151–58.

Nakatani, N. "Chemistry of Antioxidants from Labiatae Herbs." In: Huang, M. T. , T. Osawa, C. T. Ho, R. T. Rosen, eds. *Food Phytochemicals for Cancer Prevention II. Teas, Spices and Herbs.* Washington, DC: American Chemical Society, 1994: 144–53.

Ochiai, T., S. Ohno, S. Soeda, H. Tanaka, Y. Shoyama, and H. Shimeno. "Crocin Prevents the Death of Rat Pheochromyctoma (PC-12) Cells by its Antioxidant Effects Stronger Than Those of Alpha-Tocopherol." *Neuroscience Letters* 362 (May 2004): 61–64.

Pearce, B. C., R. A. Parker, M. E. Deason, A. A. Qureshi, J. J. Wright. "Hypocholesterolemic Activity of Synthetic and Natural Tocotrienols." *Journal of Medical Chemistry* 35 (1992): 3595–3606.

Phytochemical Database, USDA-ARS-NGRL, Beltsville Agricultural Research Center, Beltsville, Maryland.

Sacchetti, G., A. Medici, S. Maietti, M. Radice, M. Muzzoli, S. Manfredini, E. Braccioli, and R. Bruni. "Composition and Functional Properties of the Essential Oil of Amazonian Basil, Ocimum Micranthum Willd., Labiatae in Comparison with Commercial Essential Oils." *Journal of Agricultural and Food Chemistry* 52 (June 2004): 3486–91.

Sekiya, K., A. Ohtani, and S. Kusano. "Enhancement of Insulin Sensitivity in Adipocytes by Ginger." *Biofactors* 22 (2004): 153–56.

Verma, S. K., and A. Bordia. "Antioxidant Property of Saffron in Man." *Indian Journal of Medical Sciences* 52 (May 1998): 205–7.

Yazdanparast, R., and M. Alavi. "Antihyperlipidaemic and Antihypercholesterolaemic Effects of Anethum Graveolens Leaves After the Removal of Furocoumarins." *Cytobios* 105 (2001): 185–91.

Index